Pharmacy Registration
Assessment Questions 4

Pharmacy Registration Assessment Questions 4

Nadia Bukhari (Series Managing Editor)

BPharm, FRPharmS, FHEA, PG Dip Pharm Prac, PG Dip T&L in Higher Ed
Principal Teaching Fellow, UCL School of Pharmacy

Dr Ryan Hamilton (Contributor)

PhD, MPharm (Hons), PGDip (Clinical Pharmacy), PGCert (Independent Prescribing), MRPharmS, MFRPSI, AMRSC, AFHEA
Advanced Specialist Pharmacist in Antimicrobials, University Hospitals of Leicester NHS Trust
Honorary Senior Lecturer, School of Pharmacy, De Montfort University, Leicester

Sonia Kauser (Contributor)

PGCert (Advanced Clinical Practitioner), Independent Prescriber, PGCert (Hospital Pharmacy), MPharm, Clinical Lecturer (University of Manchester), Advanced Clinical Pharmacist Practitioner

Oksana Pyzik (Contributor)

MPharm, MRPharmS
Senior Teaching Fellow at the UCL School of Pharmacy in the Department of Practice and Policy

Pratik Thakkar (Contributor)

MPharm, MRPharmS
Medical Advisor - Oncology, Bristol-Myers Squibb

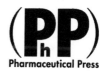
Pharmaceutical Press

Published by the Pharmaceutical Press
66-68 East Smithfield, London E1W 1AW, UK

© Pharmaceutical Press 2020

(**PP**) is a trade mark of Pharmaceutical Press

Pharmaceutical Press is the publishing division of the Royal Pharmaceutical Society

First published 2020

Typeset by SPi Global, Chennai, India
Printed in Great Britain by TJ International, Padstow, Cornwall

ISBN 978 0 85711 384 9 (print)
ISBN 978 0 85711 385 6 (kindle)
ISBN 978 0 85711 387 0 (epdf)
ISBN 978 0 85711 386 3 (ePub)

A catalogue record for this book is available from the British Library

Disclaimer
The views expressed in this book are solely those of the authors and do not necessarily reflect the views or policies of the Royal Pharmaceutical Society. This book does NOT guarantee success in the registration exam but can be used as an aid for revision.

To all the trainee pharmacists: never stop believing, never stop learning.

Nadia Bukhari 2020

Contents

Preface

After the overwhelming success of our first four volumes of *Registration Exam Questions*, a decision was made to launch a new series named *Pharmacy Registration Assessment Questions* (PRAQ). In this new series we hope to incorporate questions that are aligned to the new GPhC Framework and incorporate a similar style of questions to what has recently been announced by the GPhC for the Registration Assessment.

Both editions of volume 1 have been well received, as well as volume 2 and 3, hence encouraging the writing of a new volume.

Volume 4 of PRAQ is a bank of just under 500 questions, which are similar to the style of the registration examination. The majority of the questions are based on law and ethics, and clinical pharmacy and therapeutic aspects of the registration examination syllabus, as well as pharmaceutical calculations.

After completing 4 years of study and graduating with a Master of Pharmacy (MPharm) degree, graduates are required to undertake training as a pre-registration pharmacist before they can sit the registration examination.

Pre-registration training is the period of employment on which graduates must embark and effectively complete before they can register as a pharmacist in the UK. In most cases it is a 1-year period after the pharmacy degree; for sandwich course students it is integrated within the undergraduate programme.

On successfully passing the registration examination, pharmacy graduates can register as a pharmacist in the UK.

The registration examination harmonises the testing of skills in practice during the pre-registration year. It tests:

- knowledge
- the application of knowledge
- calculation
- time management
- managing stress
- comprehension

- recall
- interpretation
- evaluation.

There are two examination papers: Paper 1 (calculations paper with extracts) and Paper 2 (closed book paper with extracts). Questions are based on practice-based situations and are designed to test the thinking and knowledge that lie behind any action.

EXAMINATION FORMAT

The registration examination consists of two papers:

1   Paper 1: calculations with extracts

- free text answers; calculators can be used (these are not provided by GPhC)
- 40 calculations in 120 minutes (2 hours)
- extracts from reference sources provided for questions that require additional information

2   Paper 2: closed book with extracts

- multiple-choice question (MCQ) paper with extracts from reference sources provided
- 120 questions in 150 minutes (2.5 hours)

Two types of MCQs are used:

- 90 single best answer questions
- 30 extended matching questions

The registration examination is crucial for pharmacy graduates wishing to register in the UK.

Due to student demand, *Pharmacy Registration Assessment Questions* will be an annual publication with brand-new questions for students to attempt. We hope to include questions on most aspects of the examination and will take any changes made by the GPhC into consideration.

Preparation is the key. This book cannot guarantee that you will pass the registration assessment; however, it can help you to identify your learning needs and practice questions with themes and elements from within the GPhC framework questions. And, as they say, 'practice makes perfect'.

This book is written with the most current *BNF* at the time of writing. Please use the most current *BNF* and reference sources when using this book.

Good luck with the preparation and the assessment.

Nadia Bukhari
January 2020

Acknowledgements

The editor wishes to acknowledge the support from colleagues at the UCL School of Pharmacy.

Thank you to all four contributors: Ryan Hamilton, Sonia Kauser, Oksana Pyzik and Pratik Thakkar.

Nadia Bukhari would like to express thanks to the editors at Pharmaceutical Press for their support and patience in the writing of this book, and especially to Mark Pollard for his guidance.

About the authors

Nadia Bukhari BPharm, FRPharmS, FHEA, PG Dip Pharm Prac, PG Dip T&L in Higher Ed

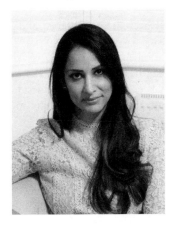

Nadia Bukhari is a Principal Teaching Fellow for Pharmacy Practice at UCL.

Her interest in writing emerged in her first year of working in academia. Seventeen years on, Nadia has authored 10 titles with the Pharmaceutical Press.

She is the Chair for the National RPS Pre-registration Conferences. She developed the extremely popular and oversubscribed conference when it first started in 2012. Nadia's outreach is wide. She has access to many young pharmacists and is accessible to them through many of her networks. In particular, via her role as an educator for pharmacy undergraduates to her position as Chair for the Royal Pharmaceutical Society national conferences, Nadia directly interacts with almost every trainee pharmacist in England. Her social media presence globalises this interaction on a huge scale.

She has a proven track record within the pharmacy profession and is the UCL Global Pharmacy Ambassador. As well as having a well-known reputation within the pharmacy profession in the UK, Nadia has also built a global reputation for herself in countries such as Pakistan, UAE, Oman, Poland, Greece, Brazil, Portugal, Italy and Belgium where she has advocated the role of the pharmacist in the UK.

Nadia has been recognised for her outstanding contributions to the profession by the pharmacy professional body, the Royal Pharmaceutical Society, and is the youngest female and youngest Asian to be awarded the status of Fellow of the Royal Pharmaceutical Society. She is the first Muslim woman to have been elected onto the National Pharmacy Board for England, which sets the strategy for the profession and influences on a government level.

Importantly, Nadia uses her platform to be vocal and prominent advocate for women's rights and is an ambassador and on the Board of Trustees for Pakistan Alliance for Girls Education (PAGE); a charity organisation supported by the government of Pakistan which promotes gender equality in education. In this advocacy role she is currently involved in a huge national project to get more girls going to school in Pakistan. In addition, she has launched the National Alliance for Women in Pharmacy in Pakistan to promote gender equity nationally for female pharmacists.

Following this, Nadia has been appointed as the Global Leader for Gender Equity at the Workforce Development hub for the International Pharmaceutical Federation (FIP).

'Leadership in Pharmacy' is Nadia's research area of interest and is currently in her final year of study for her PhD.

Nadia is a Fellow of the Higher Education Academy. Nadia is very conscientious and strives to be the best she can be. Teaching and training undergraduates and pharmacists have always been a passion and drive for Nadia. She always looks for avenues on how to excel her teaching and improve the practice of pharmacy globally.

Dr Ryan Hamilton PhD, MPharm (Hons), PGDip (Clinical Pharmacy), PGCert (Independent Prescribing), MRPharmS, MFRPSI, AMRSC, AFHEA

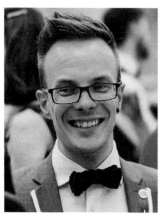

Ryan Hamilton is an Advanced Specialist Pharmacist in Antimicrobials & Acute Medicine at the University Hospitals of Leicester NHS Trust and an Honorary Senior Lecturer at the School of Pharmacy, De Montfort University, Leicester.

Ryan studied pharmacy at Liverpool John Moore's University, to which he returned after completing his pre-registration training at King's College Hospital, London, to undertake a PhD in pharmaceutical sciences. His PhD research investigated the interaction of antimicrobial agents with clay minerals and the development of candidate materials for the treatment of infected wounds. Ryan's current research focuses on the optimal use of antimicrobial agents, from antimicrobial stewardship through to use in special populations; the impact of stewardship interventions; and engagement with influenza vaccination by pharmacy professionals. He is widely published in peer-reviewed journals and professional publications and has presented his research both nationally and internationally.

Ryan also leads on antimicrobial resistance outreach projects locally and nationally, then developing a national programme to teach children and young people about infection, hygiene, antimicrobial resistance and best use of antibiotics. He also collaborates with the Leicester Media School, engaging Communication Arts students with the issues surrounding drug-resistant infections. Ryan also supports the work of Antibiotic Research UK by sitting on the charity's Education Committee.

Throughout his career Ryan has supported pharmacy students and pre-registration pharmacists. As President of the British Pharmaceutical Students' Association, he developed guidance for students and trainees, and worked closely with the GPhC to ensure trainees were fairly represented. Ryan now acts as an ambassador for the BPSA and sits on the RPS's Education and Standards Committee. Ryan has been a tutor on the RPS Pre-registration Revision and Mock Weekends for 5 years, focusing on teaching pharmaceutical calculations.

Sonia Kauser MPharm, PG Dip Hosp Pharm, PG Dip (Advanced Clinical Practitioner, Independent Prescriber)

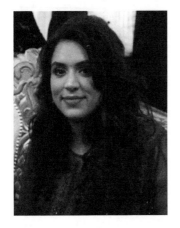

Sonia Kauser is currently a lecturer in pharmacy practice at the University of Manchester, a GP practice clinical pharmacist and an advanced clinical practitioner (minor ailments).

She began her career as a pre-registration pharmacy student at Bradford Teaching Hospitals NHS Foundation Trust and then continued her role as a hospital pharmacist. She undertook training in various specialist rotations including paediatrics, oncology, psychiatry, general medicine, surgery, anticoagulation, cardiovascular and respiratory. She was able to pursue a postgraduate diploma in Clinical Hospital Pharmacy at the University of Bradford.

Sonia then transferred her skills to primary care in which she began the role of a Clinical GP Pharmacist (based in Yorkshire). This role enabled her to pursue Level 7 Independent Prescribing and her area of specialism was initially anticoagulation. This role has now developed and she undertakes various tasks including clinical medication reviews. She predominantly works as a clinical primary care pharmacist with an interest in anticoagulation and chronic disease management. She then decided to develop her skills and attained a postgraduate diploma in Advanced Practice – Clinical Practitioner, which allows her to manage minor ailment patients within a primary care or urgent care setting. This role allows her to work and support other health care professionals (such as GPs and nurses) by triaging patients and ensuring they are signposted to the correct services. This experience in primary care has allowed her to be part of national pilots for extended access/out of hours schemes.

Sonia has also worked in the following areas: urgent care, out of hours (walk-in centre), GSK (training of pharmaceutical reps), community pharmacy, acute ward pharmacist at Leeds Teaching Hospitals and guest lecturer role at the University of Bradford.

Sonia enjoys keeping active, reading and shopping in her spare time. Her most recent publication was in the *Prescriber Journal* June 2017 and describes the use of clinical information systems to improve practice within primary care.

Oksana Pyzik MPharm, MRPharmS

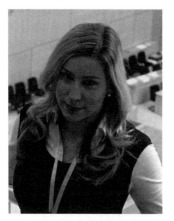

Oksana Pyzik is a Senior Teaching Fellow and Global Engagement Coordinator at University College London (UCL) School of Pharmacy. In addition to her role in education, Oksana is also a Global Health Advisor and Board Trustee of the Commonwealth Pharmacists Association. Oksana first started her career as a pharmacist in the primary care setting delivering public health interventions to marginalised patient groups in underserved communities across London. It was this early experience in practice that motivated her to conduct public health research at the International Pharmaceutical Federation (FIP) before moving into the academic sector full time in 2013. She went on to earn her Post Graduate Diploma in Teaching and Learning in Higher Professional Education at the Institute of Education in 2015 and is now a Fellow of the UK Higher Education Academy. In 2017, Oksana was appointed as the FIP UCL FIPEd Collaborating Centre Global Engagement Liaison in recognition of her leadership within pharmacy and global health. Oksana is extensively involved with the Royal Pharmaceutical Society (RPS) Preregistration Conferences in both the development of teaching material and the delivery of training sessions. She also remains active in community pharmacy setting, serving as the Preregistration and Academic Lead for the Central London Local Practice Forum (LPF) where she acts as a link between community pharmacy and academia in this role.

Pratik Thakkar MPharm, MRPharmS

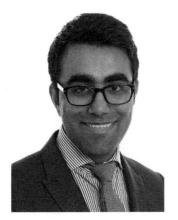

Pratik Thakkar graduated from UCL School of Pharmacy and completed his preregistration placement at Great Ormond Street Hospital for Children.

After qualifying, he continued to work at Great Ormond Street as a Parenteral Nutrition and Quality Assurance Pharmacist. Following this, Pratik took an opportunity to work at the Medicines and Healthcare products Regulatory Agency (MHRA) in London in the Vigilance and Risk Management of Medicines department to gain further knowledge in pharmacovigilance (PV) and Regulatory Affairs.

He has also worked at Mylan Inc. in Product Safety and Risk Management. He was a PV pharmacist in the Global Pharmacovigilance function, as well as in Medical Affairs. He worked on various projects to monitor the safety of the company's products on the market, as well as working on signing off material in line with the UK and Ireland Codes of Practice.

Pratik now works at Bristol-Myers Squibb where he has held various posts within Medical Governance and Compliance and Medical Affairs. He has gained experience in rheumatology and now oncology as a Medical Advisor. He has attained ABPI and IPHA final signatory status for the UK and Irish business. He is actively involved in developing medical strategy for various oncology therapy indications and working closely with cross-functional teams and within the company to deliver innovative medicines for patients with serious and life-threatening diseases.

Abbreviations

ACBS	Advisory Committee on Borderline Substances
ACE	angiotensin-converting enzyme
ACEI	angiotensin-converting enzyme inhibitor
ACS	acute coronary syndrome
AF	atrial fibrillation
ALT DIE	alternate days
AV	arteriovenous
BD	twice daily
BMI	body mass index
BNF	*British National Formulary*
BNFC	*British National Formulary for Children*
BP	blood pressure
BPSA	British Pharmaceutical Students' Association
BSA	body surface area
BTS	British Thoracic Society
CCF	congestive/chronic cardiac failure
CD	controlled drug
CDC	US Centers for Disease Control and Prevention
CE	*conformité européenne*
CFC	chlorofluorocarbon
CHM	Commission on Human Medicines
CHMP	Committee for Medicinal Products for Human Use
CI	confidence interval or cumulative incidence
CKS	Clinical Knowledge Summaries
COX	cyclooxygenase
COPD	chronic obstructive pulmonary disease
CPD	continuing professional development
CPPE	Centre for Pharmacy Postgraduate Education
CrCl	creatinine clearance (mL/min)
CSM	Committee on Safety of Medicines
CYT	cytochrome
DigCl	digoxin clearance (L/h)

DMARD	disease-modifying antirheumatic drug
DNG	discount not given
DPF	*Dental Practitioners' Formulary*
DPI	dry-powder inhaler
EC	enteric-coated
ECG	electrocardiogram
EEA	European Economic Area
eGFR	estimated glomerular filtration rate
EHC	emergency hormonal contraception
F1	Foundation Year 1
FEV_1	forced expiratory volume in 1 second
GP	general practitioner
GP6D	glucose-6-phosphate dehydrogenase
GPhC	General Pharmaceutical Council
GSL	general sales list
GTN	glyceryl trinitrate
HbA1c	glycated haemoglobin
HDU	high dependency unit
HIV	human immunodeficiency virus
HR	heart rate
HRT	hormone replacement therapy
IBS	irritable bowel syndrome
IBW	ideal body weight
IDA	industrial denatured alcohol
IM	intramuscular
INR	international normalised ratio
IV	intravenous
IUD	intrauterine device
MAOI	monoamine oxidase inhibitor
MD	maximum single dose
MDD	maximum daily dose
MDI	metered-dose inhaler
MDU	to be used as directed
MEP	*Medicines, Ethics and Practice* guide
MHRA	Medicines and Healthcare products Regulatory Agency
MMR	measles, mumps and rubella
M/R	modified-release
MRSA	methicillin-resistant *Staphylococcus aureus*
MUPS	multiple-unit pellet system
MUR	Medicines Use Review

NHS	National Health Service
NICE	National Institute for Health and Care Excellence
NMS	New Medicines Service
NRLS	National Reporting and Learning System
NSAIDs	non-steroidal anti-inflammatory drugs
OC	oral contraceptive
OD	*omni die* (every day)
OM	*omni mane* (every morning)
ON	*omni nocte* (every night)
OP	original pack
OPAT	outpatient parenteral antibacterial therapy
ORT	oral rehydration therapy
OTC	over-the-counter
P	pharmacy
PAGB	Proprietary Association of Great Britain
PCT	primary care trust
PHE	Public Health England
PIL	patient information leaflet
pMDI	pressurised metered-dose inhaler
PMR	patient medical record
POM	prescription-only medicine
POM-V	prescription-only medicine – veterinarian
POM-VPS	prescription-only medicine – veterinarian, pharmacist, suitably qualified person
PPIs	proton pump inhibitors
PRN	when required
PSA	prostate-specific antigen
PSNC	Pharmaceutical Services Negotiating Committee
QDS	*quarter die sumendum* (to be taken four times daily)
RCT	randomised controlled trial
RE	right eye
RPS	Royal Pharmaceutical Society (formerly RPSGB)
SARSS	Suspected Adverse Reaction Surveillance Scheme
SCRIPT	Standard Computerised Revalidation Instrument for Prescribing and Therapeutics
SeCr	serum creatinine
SGLT2	sodium (Na^+)/glucose co-transporter 2
SHO	senior house officer
SIGN	Scottish Intercollegiate Guidelines Network
SLS	selected list scheme

SOP	standard operating procedure
SPC	summary of product characteristics
SSRI	selective serotonin reuptake inhibitor
ST	an isoelectric line after the QRS complex of an ECG
STAT	immediately
TCA	tricyclic antidepressant
TDS	three times a day
TIA	transient ischaemic attack
TPN	total parenteral nutrition
TSDA	trade-specific denatured alcohol
U&E	urea and electrolyte count
UTI	urinary tract infection
VITAL	Virtual Interactive Teaching And Learning
WHO	World Health Organization

How to use this book

The book is divided into three main sections: single best answer questions, extended matching questions and calculation questions.

SINGLE BEST ANSWER QUESTIONS (SBAs)

Each of the questions or statements in this section is followed by five suggested answers. Select the best answer in each situation.

For example:
A patient on your ward has been admitted with a gastric ulcer, which is currently being treated. She has a history of arthritis and cardiac problems. Which of her drugs is most likely to have caused the gastric ulcer?

- ☐ A   Paracetamol
- ☐ B   Naproxen
- ☐ C   Furosemide
- ☐ D   Propranolol
- ☐ E   Codeine phosphate

EXTENDED MATCHING QUESTIONS (EMQs)

Extended matching questions consist of lettered options followed by a list of numbered problems/questions. For each numbered problem/question, select the one lettered option that most closely answers the question. You can use the lettered options once, more than once or not at all.

For example:
Antidepressants

- A   Amitriptyline
- B   Citalopram
- C   Duloxetine
- D   Flupentixol

E   Mirtazapine
F   Moclobemide
G   St John's wort
H   Venlafaxine

For questions 1–4
For the patients described, select the single most likely antidepressant from the list above. Each option may be used once, more than once or not at all.

1   Miss K is a 32-year-old woman on your ward who has a long-standing history of depression related to her chronic illness. She has tried antidepressants in the past but stopped them when she felt better. The medical team tell you that she returns to hospital periodically with relapsed symptoms because she stops taking her medicines. They want to treat her depression but the agent they suggest would not be suitable for Miss K, considering her non-adherence.

2   One of the new GPs in the surgery across the road calls you for some advice. He has a patient with him, Mr B, who is 28 years old and has agreed to try an antidepressant medicine. Mr B is otherwise fit and healthy, but the GP would like your advice on what to prescribe for this new diagnosis of moderate depression.

3   Three months later you get another call from the GP about Mr B, who has not responded well to the initial antidepressants and may be experiencing a number of side-effects. They want to switch him on to a different agent quickly, if not immediately. You inform the GP that one of the drugs he asked about cannot be started immediately.

4   Mrs C has just been admitted on to your emergency admissions unit after being referred directly from her GP, whom she went to see about her headache. On admission she also complains of palpitations and her BP is 205/100 mmHg. On taking her history you note she is Japanese and still eats a traditional diet, leading you to suspect her antidepressant medicine may have precipitated this condition.

CALCULATION QUESTIONS

These are free text pharmaceutical calculations. The use of calculators is permitted when tackling these questions. The GPhC will provide candidates with calculators for the purpose of the assessment.

For example:

Mrs D is a 75-year-old woman who has just been admitted to your respiratory ward with an exacerbation of asthma. On admission she was weighed at 97 kg and states her height as 5 feet 3 inches. When taking her history, you find she quit smoking 10 years ago and is on the following medicines:

- Fostair 100/6 two puffs BD
- Budesonide 4 mg PO OM
- *Phyllocontin Continus* (aminophylline) 225-mg tablets, two tablets BD MDU
- Salbutamol 2.5 mg nebulised QDS PRN
- Salbutamol 100-mcg CFC-free inhaler 2–6 puffs QDS PRN via an aerochamber (blue)

How much aminophylline should Mrs D receive over the next 24 hours? Give your answer to the nearest whole number.

> The purpose of the registration assessment is to test a candidate's ability to apply the knowledge they have learnt over the past five years of their education and training.
>
> Testing someone's ability to locate information efficiently in the *BNF* should be tested during their pre-registration training year and in their undergraduate training.
>
> Therefore, all questions are closed book, with extracts of reference sources provided to candidates.

Answers to the questions are at the end of the book. Brief explanations or a suitable reference for sourcing the answer are given, to aid understanding and to facilitate learning.

Important: this text refers to the current edition of the *BNF* and *BNFC* when text was written. Please always consult the LATEST version for the most up-to-date information.

Single best answer questions

Sonia Kauser

1   Miss JS, aged 38, visits the community pharmacy and requests beclometasone nasal spray. She informs you she has a history of allergic rhinitis and also suffers from seasonal allergy. She has been advised to use this spray but is unsure how long she can use the spray for. She has no known other medical conditions and no known drug allergies. You decide to supply the spray and explain the maximum usage.
What is the recommended maximum duration of the nasal spray?

    ☐ A   7 days
    ☐ B   14 days
    ☐ C   1 month
    ☐ D   2 months
    ☐ E   3 months

2   Mrs GB, aged 32, has visited the community pharmacy seeking advice regarding her daughter, OJ who is 6 years old. After reviewing her symptoms, you decide she needs to be treated with mebendazole due to a diagnosis of threadworm.
Which of the following statements is correct regarding mebendazole?

    ☐ A   If you are re-infected, it may be appropriate to take a further course after 2 weeks
    ☐ B   It is recommended to treat all family members who are infected
    ☐ C   It is suitable to provide this to pregnant patients
    ☐ D   Mebendazole is licensed in children over the age of 1 year
    ☐ E   Treatment is usually once daily over a course of 7 days

3   Mr TS, aged 29, presents to the pharmacy with a red eye. He has not previously experienced these symptoms and woke up this morning with a red left eye. He would like your advice. On examining the eye, you note redness on the area of the left eye. The right eye is unaffected. Mr TS reports nil pain and nil discharge. He does not have a temperature and states he feels fit and well otherwise.
What is the likely diagnosis?

    □ **A**   Bacterial conjunctivitis
    □ **B**   Haemorrhagic conjunctivitis
    □ **C**   Keratitis
    □ **D**   Subconjunctival haemorrhage
    □ **E**   Viral conjunctivitis

4   Mr CK, aged 52, presents to the pharmacy requesting *Sudafed*® tablets. Upon questioning you note that he has taken this medication in the past for a blocked nose and he found it useful in clearing his symptoms.
Which of the following statements is correct regarding *Sudafed*®?

    □ **A**   The active ingredient in each tablet is pseudoephedrine 6 mg
    □ **B**   This medication is for the use in adults and children aged 12 years and above
    □ **C**   This medication is safe to use in diabetes
    □ **D**   This medication is safe to use in hypertension
    □ **E**   This medication is used for blocked noses, sinuses, runny nose, catarrh and epistaxis

5   Mr GF, aged 22, visits the pharmacy with a concern regarding pain when opening his bowels. You decide to discuss his symptoms with him, and he informs you the pain occurs whilst his bowels move. He has also noticed a small speck of fresh blood upon wiping. He was constipated 1 week ago but this has now resolved. He has not experienced these symptoms in the past.
Which of the following is the most appropriate way to manage Mr GF?

    □ **A**   Manage with *AnuSol*® ointment
    □ **B**   Manage with ibuprofen gel 5%
    □ **C**   Manage with 1 g glyceryl suppositories PR
    □ **D**   Refer to A & E
    □ **E**   Refer to GP

6   Which of the following medications should be prescribed and dispensed by brand due to differences in bioavailability between various formulations?

      ☐ **A**   Amlodipine
      ☐ **B**   Aripiprazole
      ☐ **C**   Fluoxetine
      ☐ **D**   Hyoscine butylbromide
      ☐ **E**   Tacrolimus

7   Miss SK, aged 55, presents to the community pharmacy wanting some advice regarding her pain relief medication. She recently purchased ibuprofen 400 mg tablets 2 days ago and has been experiencing pain in her abdomen and noticed dark stools when she visited the toilet. She is unsure how to proceed.
Which of the following is the most appropriate recommendation?

      ☐ **A**   Reassure patient and advise to continue with ibuprofen
      ☐ **B**   Refer to A & E
      ☐ **C**   Refer to GP to issue a proton pump inhibitor
      ☐ **D**   Stop ibuprofen and wait 24 hours for symptoms to resolve
      ☐ **E**   Stop ibuprofen, replace with paracetamol and wait 24 hours for symptoms to resolve

8   Mr DF, aged 48, visits the pharmacy with a localised rash on his left arm. Upon examining you note that there is a red round circular presentation. There is a sharp margin and raised edges. Mr DF explains it is quite itchy and has been present for 2 days.
What is the most appropriate way to manage Mr DF?

      ☐ **A**   Refer to A & E
      ☐ **B**   Refer to GP
      ☐ **C**   Supply clobetasone butyrate 0.05% cream
      ☐ **D**   Supply miconazole 2% powder
      ☐ **E**   Supply OTC clotrimazole 1% cream

9   Mr DG, aged 48, presents to the pharmacy requesting management of a lesion on his foot. Mr DG takes the following medication: ramipril 5 mg OD, paracetamol 1 g QDS, atorvastatin 80 mg ON, aspirin 75 mg OD, bisoprolol 5 mg OD, metformin 500 mg TDS, glimepiride 2 mg OD and lansoprazole 15 mg OD.
Upon examining the lesion, you note tiny black dots collected under the surface of hard skin. The lesion is approximately 5 mm wide.
What is the most appropriate way to manage this patient?

      ☐ **A**   Refer to GP
      ☐ **B**   Supply *Bazuka*™ gel
      ☐ **C**   Supply *Iglu*® gel

    ☐ **D**   Supply 1% clotrimazole cream
    ☐ **E**   Supply 2% miconazole cream

10 Mrs KF, aged 32, presents with her 18-month-old daughter, Miss SM, due to a query related to her eye. Miss SM woke up this morning with a sticky right eye. She is in no pain; however, Mrs KF has noticed Miss SM rubbing her eyes on waking. The yellow discharge is purulent and unilateral.
What is the most appropriate way to manage Mrs KF?

    ☐ **A**   Refer to GP
    ☐ **B**   Supply OTC chloramphenicol 0.5% eye drops for a 5-day course
    ☐ **C**   Supply OTC chloramphenicol 0.5% eye drops for a 7-day course
    ☐ **D**   Supply OTC chloramphenicol 1% eye ointment for a 5-day course
    ☐ **E**   Supply OTC chloramphenicol 1% eye ointment for a 7-day course

11 You are a community-based pharmacist and receive a call from the local GP within the health centre you work at. The query is related to a known patient – Mrs GF, aged 72, who has known chronic pain. She is unable to tolerate a higher dose of her fentanyl patch (she is currently prescribed a 37.5 microgram patch applied every 72 hours). The GP is considering the addition of a buprenorphine patch to help with pain management.
What advice do you give to the GP?

    ☐ **A**   Avoid the addition of buprenorphine patch as it will cause addiction
    ☐ **B**   Avoid the addition of buprenorphine patch as it will increase the risk of opiate withdrawal
    ☐ **C**   Can add buprenorphine but recommend an alternative route such as sublingual tablets
    ☐ **D**   Can add buprenorphine patch at any strength due to patient's history of chronic pain
    ☐ **E**   Can add buprenorphine patch at the lowest strength possible and titrate up

12 Miss FN, aged 28, has been prescribed *Roaccutane*® PO for her severe acne by her specialist. She presents with a prescription to the community pharmacy and this is the initial dispensing of this prescription.

Which of the following is correct advice regarding this medication?

   ☐ A   It is safe to fall pregnant whilst taking this medication

   ☐ B   Monitoring requirements include full blood count and urea and electrolytes

   ☐ C   Patients with a history of depression do not require close supervision

   ☐ D   This medication can cause increased libido

   ☐ E   This medication is prescribed based on patient weight

13 Miss GH, aged 26, presents to the community pharmacy with an FP10 prescription for *Roaccutane*®.
How long is this prescription valid for?

   ☐ A   7 days

   ☐ B   14 days

   ☐ C   28 days

   ☐ D   6 months

   ☐ E   Not NHS prescribable

14 Mr MS, aged 62, has attended for his annual health check at the GP surgery. You are the pharmacist working at the practice and note his QRISK3 score is 11%. You review his medication and note he is prescribed the following: rivaroxaban 20 mg OD (atrial fibrillation history), bisoprolol 5 mg OD (atrial fibrillation history), lansoprazole 15 mg OD (acid reflux history).
Which of the following statements is correct regarding his risk score?

   ☐ A   This patient is already anticoagulated therefore no further review needed

   ☐ B   This patient is already prescribed a proton pump inhibitor for gastroprotection therefore no further review is needed

   ☐ C   This patient is at a high risk of a cardiovascular event therefore requires a discussion regarding initiation of new medication

   ☐ D   This patient is at a high risk of a cardiovascular event therefore requires a discussion regarding lifestyle modification

   ☐ E   This patient is at a low risk of a cardiovascular event therefore no further action needed

15 Mr AJ, aged 58, has been recently diagnosed with osteoporosis. You are reviewing his recent bone density scan at the general practice surgery you work for. The recommendation is to start bisphosphonate therapy.

Which of the following is an appropriate recommendation?

☐ **A** Alendronic acid 70 mg daily
☐ **B** Alendronic acid 70 mg once weekly
☐ **C** Risedronate 5 mg once daily
☐ **D** Risedronate 35 mg once daily
☐ **E** Risedronate 35 mg once weekly

16 Mr FN, aged 73, has a CHA2DS2-VASc score of 2. His current medications are as follows: amlodipine 5 mg OD, sertraline 50 mg OD, *Clenil*® 100 mcg inhale 1 puff BD, salbutamol 100 mcg inhale 1 puff PRN.
What do you recommend as the appropriate course of action?

☐ **A** Discuss the initiation of aspirin therapy
☐ **B** Discuss the initiation of atorvastatin therapy
☐ **C** Discuss the initiation of warfarin therapy
☐ **D** When the score reaches 3 then consider discussing medication prevention therapy
☐ **E** When the score reaches 4 then consider discussing medication prevention therapy

17 Mr BH, aged 29, is prescribed metronidazole from his dentist. He presents to the community pharmacy with a prescription stating 400 mg TDS.
Which of the following statements is correct?

☐ **A** Doses do not need to be spaced evenly throughout the day
☐ **B** Drinking alcohol is safe to do so with this medication
☐ **C** Tablets can be crushed or chewed for administration
☐ **D** Take with half a glass of water
☐ **E** Take with or after food

18 Mrs SR, aged 52, visits the pharmacy and mentions she may be due for a routine mammogram test. She has no history of breast cancer and no family history of breast cancer.
What do you advise?

☐ **A** No test recommended as there is no history of breast cancer
☐ **B** Routine test every year is recommended
☐ **C** Routine test every 2 years is recommended
☐ **D** Routine test every 3 years is recommended
☐ **E** Routine test every 4 years is recommended

19 Which of the following antidepressant medications is associated with the LEAST withdrawal side effects if stopped abruptly?

- ☐ A   Citalopram 10 mg OD
- ☐ B   Escitalopram 20 mg OD
- ☐ C   Fluoxetine 20 mg OD
- ☐ D   Paroxetine 20 mg OD
- ☐ E   Paroxetine 40 mg OD

20 Which of the following antidepressant medications is associated with weight gain as a common side effect?

- ☐ A   Amitriptyline
- ☐ B   Citalopram
- ☐ C   Escitalopram
- ☐ D   Lofepramine
- ☐ E   Mirtazapine

21 Which of the following medications would require liver function monitoring at regular 3-monthly intervals if treatment is required for longer than 6 months?

- ☐ A   Duloxetine
- ☐ B   Griseofulvin
- ☐ C   Levofloxacin
- ☐ D   Minocycline
- ☐ E   Simvastatin

22 Mrs FK, aged 65, visits your community pharmacy for a routine prescription for citalopram 30 mg daily. Her comorbidities include COPD and hypertension. She has been taking citalopram for many years and upon discussing this medication with her, she informs you she intends to continue taking this for at least a further year.
Which of the following is the most appropriate advice for Mrs FK?

- ☐ A   She can continue as she has been stable for many years
- ☐ B   To book in for a medicines use review in 1 years' time to discuss the citalopram again
- ☐ C   To speak to her GP to consider increasing the dose to 40 mg daily
- ☐ D   To speak to her GP to discuss amending to escitalopram 10 mg daily
- ☐ E   To speak to her GP to discuss reducing the dose to 20 mg daily

23 Mr MK, aged 32, has been initiated on naproxen therapy for his pain relief as he has rheumatoid arthritis. The GP has prescribed him naproxen 500 mg BD PRN. He presents to the community pharmacy with his prescription. His current medication is as follows: sertraline 100 mg OD, salbutamol 100 mg inhale 2 puffs PRN, *Fostair*® 100/6 1 puff BD, paracetamol 1g QDS.
Which of the following is the most appropriate advice to give to the GP?

  □ A Consider adding in a proton pump inhibitor
  □ B Consider amending naproxen to the gastro-resistant formulation
  □ C Consider monitoring urea and electrolytes due to raised potassium risk
  □ D Consider reducing dose to 250 mg BD as this is his first prescription
  □ E Consider reducing dose to 250 mg every 6–8 hours as this is his first prescription

24 Miss TH, aged 33, has been initiated on a medication which requires routine weight monitoring due to an increased risk of weight gain.
Which of the following will be the likely medication?

  □ A Aripiprazole
  □ B Olanzapine
  □ C Zuclopenthixol
  □ D All the above
  □ E None of the above

25 Mr FR, aged 29, has been initiated on lithium therapy for his bipolar affective disorder. A normal drug range level is 0.4–1 mmol/L.
When should a drug sample be taken to ensure the correct range is determined?

  □ A 6 hours post dose
  □ B 8 hours post dose
  □ C 10 hours post dose
  □ D 12 hours post dose
  □ E 24 hours post dose

26 Mrs EB, aged 74, is admitted to the local hospital due to suspected digoxin toxicity. Her current medication is as follows: digoxin 125 mcg OD, bisoprolol 1.25 mg OD, simvastatin 20 mg ON, clopidogrel 75 mg OD, alendronic acid 70 mg once weekly, *Calceos*® 1 BD.

Which of the following statements is correct with regards to digoxin monitoring?

☐ A   Digoxin drug level ranges are usually 0.4–1 mcg/L
☐ B   Routine digoxin drug levels are not recommended
☐ C   Routine digoxin drug levels are only recommended in elderly patients
☐ D   Routine digoxin drug levels are recommended in all high-risk patients
☐ E   The bioavailability does not change when converting from tablets to liquid

27   Mrs CM, aged 58, has recently had an exacerbation of her COPD. She is a known patient at your community pharmacy and presents with the following prescription: amoxicillin 500 mg TDS, prednisolone 30 mg OD for 7 days. You check her PMR and note the following repeat medication: seretide 250 evohaler inhale 2 puffs BD, tiotriopum 18 mcg inhale 1 puff OD, risedronate 35 mg OD, *Adcal-D₃*® chewable 1 BD, ramipril 5 mg OD, furosemide 20 mg OD, bisoprolol 1.25 mg OD, atorvastatin 20 mg OD. Her acute medication is as follows: co-codamol 15/500 mg 2 QDS PRN issued 1 month ago, prednisolone 5 mg OD stopped 11 months ago.

Which of the following statements is correct regarding her current prescription?

☐ A   Consider a gradual reduction dose over a longer period of time
☐ B   The dose should be prednisolone 30 mg OD for 10 days
☐ C   The dose should be prednisolone 30 mg OD for 14 days
☐ D   The dose should be prednisolone 40 mg OD for 7 days
☐ E   The dose should be prednisolone 40 mg OD for 10 days

28   Miss SN, aged 32, presents to the community pharmacy with her 3-year-old son. She is concerned about a cough he developed overnight. Upon discussing the cough, you are able to note that it started 6 hours ago, there is a sudden temperature, the cough sounds like a barking cough and a hoarse voice (her son started with a runny nose 24 hours ago). There is no phlegm described by mum.

Which of the following is the most appropriate advice to give to the child's mum?

☐ A   Offer paracetamol liquid
☐ B   Offer paracetamol liquid and simple linctus paediatrics
☐ C   Offer simple linctus paediatrics
☐ D   Signpost to A & E
☐ E   Signpost to GP

29 Mr BK, aged 35, presents to the community pharmacy complaining about an earache in his right ear. He informs you it feels blocked but also is quite itchy. You confirm his past medical history which is nil medication and nil allergies. He also informs you he swims regularly to keep active.
    Which of the following is the most appropriate course of action?

  □ **A**   Offer acetic acid ear spray
  □ **B**   Offer hydrogen peroxide ear drops
  □ **C**   Offer olive oil ear drops
  □ **D**   Refer to A & E
  □ **E**   Refer to GP

30 You are a prescribing pharmacist working in a general practice environment. You are reviewing a patient (Mr BP, aged 39) at your clinic today and diagnose him with an acute exacerbation of gout. The patient did have their uric acids levels recently tested which were raised. You decide to initiate them on allopurinol therapy.
    Which of the following statements is correct regarding allopurinol?

  □ **A**   Can only be initiated by a specialist
  □ **B**   Dose adjusted according to potassium levels
  □ **C**   Dose adjusted according to sodium levels
  □ **D**   Dose usually initiated at 450 mg OD
  □ **E**   Increased risk of acute gout arthritis attack in early stages

31 Mr ZN, aged 38, is prescribed aripiprazole at a dose of 10 mg OD by his mental health specialist as he has a known history of schizophrenia. He is currently taking no other medication.
    Which of the following is the correct annual monitoring requirements for Mr ZN?

  □ **A**   Annual physical health assessment including cardiovascular risk assessment
  □ **B**   Annual prolactin
  □ **C**   Annual weight and HbA1c
  □ **D**   All the above
  □ **E**   None of the above

32 Mr SC, aged 39, has been initiated on clozapine therapy for the management of his treatment-resistant schizophrenia. As part of his treatment plan, he has been advised that he will need regular blood tests every week for the first 18 weeks, then at least every 2 weeks, and if clozapine is decided to continue long term then regular bloods at least every 4 weeks.

What of the following conditions is the monitoring required for?

- ☐ **A** Cardiomyopathy
- ☐ **B** Hyperprolactinaemia
- ☐ **C** Myocarditis
- ☐ **D** Neutropenia
- ☐ **E** Pancreatitis

33 Mrs GB, aged 42, presents to the community pharmacy with her new prescription for the following items: alendronic acid 70 mg once weekly PO, *Calceos*® 1 BD PO. She explains to you that she has not been given any counselling with her GP as they did not have enough time during her consultation. She informs you that she has been diagnosed with osteoporosis.
Which of the following statements is correct regarding her counselling?

- ☐ **A** Alendronic acid can be taken whilst standing, sitting or laying
- ☐ **B** Alendronic acid to be taken once weekly on any alternating day of the week
- ☐ **C** Avoid taking alendronic acid at the same time as *Calceos*®
- ☐ **D** She needs to continue; alendronic acid treatment will be assessed after 10 years
- ☐ **E** Take alendronic acid on a full stomach after food to prevent GI-related side effects

34 Mrs MS, aged 72, presents to your minor ailment clinic complaining of urinary symptoms. You are a prescribing pharmacist and undertake the relevant investigations including temperature (38°C), urine dipstick (positive for nitrates and leucocytes) and understanding the patient's general symptoms (dysuria, increased frequency). After reviewing the patient, you decide she does have an uncomplicated UTI. Her medication is as follows: aspirin 75 mg OD, bisoprolol 2.5 mg OD, lisinopril 10 mg OD, atorvastatin 80 mg OD, methotrexate 10 mg once weekly, folic acid 5 mg once weekly, paracetamol 1g QDS PRN, GTN spray 400 mcg S/L PRN.
Which of the following antibiotics would NOT be an appropriate treatment to consider?

- ☐ **A** Amoxicillin
- ☐ **B** Fosfomycin
- ☐ **C** Nitrofurantoin
- ☐ **D** Pivmecillinam
- ☐ **E** Trimethoprim

35 Mrs LS, aged 42, visits your pharmacy to collect her medication. She has recently been prescribed levothyroxine 50 mcg once daily for her hypothyroidism. She is currently taking no other medication.
Which of the following piece of advice is correct regarding her new medication?

    ☐ **A**   Take 30 minutes after other medication
    ☐ **B**   Take at least 30 minutes after breakfast
    ☐ **C**   Take at least 30 minutes before caffeine-containing liquid
    ☐ **D**   This medication should be taken at night
    ☐ **E**   None of the above

36 You are a community pharmacist working in a busy store within a large retail setting. You decide to add posters in the pharmacy as part of your campaign to promote smear testing. One of your regular patients, Miss FG, aged 28 years, notices the poster and asks you how often she will be required to undertake this test?
Which of the following is correct?

    ☐ **A**   Every 1 year until aged 50
    ☐ **B**   Every 2 years until aged 50
    ☐ **C**   Every 3 years until aged 50
    ☐ **D**   Every 4 years until aged 50
    ☐ **E**   Every 5 years until aged 50

37 Miss KL, aged 26, has been prescribed *Yasmin*® tablets for contraception. She has been taking this medication for the last 12 months. She currently has no contraindications to this medication.
Which of the following changes to Miss KL's health would warrant a referral to the GP?

    ☐ **A**   BMI >28 kg/m^2
    ☐ **B**   BP increases to 140/90
    ☐ **C**   Migraine with aura
    ☐ **D**   Miss KL stops smoking
    ☐ **E**   Missed pill at the beginning of the cycle

38 Mrs SB, aged 59, is currently taking hormone replacement therapy (HRT) medication (1 mg estradiol + 1 mg norethisterone) to help manage her menopausal symptoms. She informs you she is aware of the risks associated with HRT therapy but has been advised there are also benefits in taking this medication.
Which of the following is a benefit of taking HRT?

    ☐ **A**   Reduces bone fracture risk
    ☐ **B**   Reduces breast cancer risk
    ☐ **C**   Reduces ovarian cancer risk

☐ **D**   Reduces stroke risk
☐ **E**   Reduces thromboembolism risk

39   Miss FR, aged 34, has known polycystic ovary syndrome (PCOS). She is a regular patient at your community pharmacy and was hoping you could advise her on medication which may improve the symptoms of her PCOS.
What would be the most appropriate medication to suggest?

☐ **A**   Combined hormonal contraceptive pill
☐ **B**   Combined hormone replacement therapy
☐ **C**   Oestrogen-only hormone replacement therapy
☐ **D**   Progestogen-only contraceptive pill
☐ **E**   Progestogen-only hormone replacement therapy

40   Miss HC, aged 33, visits your community pharmacy complaining of acute diarrhoea. She explains she has had these symptoms for 12 hours and previously loperamide has been very helpful in stopping her diarrhoea. She is otherwise fit and well and there are no signs of dehydration. She is not taking any other medication.
Which of the following statements is correct with regards to the OTC dose for loperamide 2 mg capsules?

☐ **A**   Max 2 per day
☐ **B**   Max 4 per day
☐ **C**   Max 6 per day
☐ **D**   Max 8 per day
☐ **E**   Max 10 per day

41   Miss PL, aged 33, visits your pharmacy with a prescription for: medroxyprogesterone acetate 5 mg tablets – take one daily for 7 days then repeat for 2 cycles. She informs you the prescription is for her dysfunctional uterine bleeding.
Which of the following statements is INCORRECT regarding this medication?

☐ **A**   Avoid in those with susceptibility to thromboembolism
☐ **B**   Can be prescribed safely in patients with a history of breast cancer
☐ **C**   Can be used as a form of contraception when given by intramuscular injection
☐ **D**   Can be used as a form of contraception when given subcutaneously
☐ **E**   Non-oral route can delay fertility

42 Miss AB, aged 24, presents to your community pharmacy requesting medication to help with a headache that has lasted over 24 hours. Upon discussing her symptoms, you note it is a unilateral pulsating headache causing pain and affecting her studies. She thinks caffeine may have triggered this and has also noted she is feeling nauseous. Her past medical history includes asthma. Upon reviewing, you suspect Miss AB has a migraine and proceed to consider her analgesia options.
Which of the following statements is INCORRECT regarding her over-the-counter analgesia options?

 ☐ **A** Miss AB can be offered over-the-counter co-codamol tablets
 ☐ **B** Miss AB can be offered over-the-counter paracetamol tablets
 ☐ **C** Miss AB cannot be offered ibuprofen tablets
 ☐ **D** Miss AB cannot be offered rizatriptan due to license
 ☐ **E** Miss AB cannot be offered sumatriptan as a doctor has not yet made a formal diagnosis

43 Mrs NB presents to the community pharmacy with her 5-year-old daughter and she is concerned about a rash. You examine the patient (Miss OB) and note she has red sores around her nose and mouth. Some of the skin lesions have a golden crust and Miss OB describes the area as being itchy. Mrs NB also suspects a temperature.
Which of the following statements is correct for managing Miss OB?

 ☐ **A** Advise this is self-limiting and will disappear in 2 weeks
 ☐ **B** Refer to A & E
 ☐ **C** Refer to GP
 ☐ **D** Supply 1% clotrimazole cream
 ☐ **E** Supply aciclovir 5% cream

44 Mrs SF, aged 34, is prescribed metoclopramide for the management of radiotherapy-induced nausea and vomiting. She presents to the hospital outpatient pharmacy with her prescription.
Which of the following statements is correct regarding metoclopramide?

 ☐ **A** Avoid in acute migraine patients
 ☐ **B** Avoid in palliative care
 ☐ **C** Max 5 days use
 ☐ **D** Max daily oral dose is 40 mg
 ☐ **E** There is a low risk for inducing acute dystonic reactions

45 Mrs MT, aged 59, has been initiated on empaglifozin 10 mg OD therapy after her recent diabetes review. Her other antidiabetic medication includes metformin 500 mg TDS and glimepiride 3 mg OD.

Which of the following is an important counselling point for Mrs MT's new medication?

- ☐ **A** Increased risk of hyperglycaemia therefore monitor blood glucose
- ☐ **B** Increased risk of lactic acidosis therefore be aware of signs and symptoms
- ☐ **C** Refer to GP as NICE do not recommend triple therapy
- ☐ **D** Risk of diabetic ketoacidosis therefore be aware of signs and symptoms
- ☐ **E** All the above

46 Miss KJ, aged 25, visits your community pharmacy complaining of a local rash on her lower lip. Initially she noticed a tingling sensation which then led to a burning and tingling feeling which has lasted over 24 hours. She informs you she takes no regular medication and has no known drug allergies.
How do you manage Miss KJ?

- ☐ **A** Offer aciclovir 5% cream
- ☐ **B** Offer clotrimazole 1% cream
- ☐ **C** Offer hydrocortisone 1% cream
- ☐ **D** Offer miconazole 2% / hydrocortisone 1% cream
- ☐ **E** Refer to GP

47 You are working in general practice as a minor ailment pharmacist. Master AB (5 years old) presents to the clinic with his mum complaining of shortness of breath. His mum informs you he recently had a viral upper respiratory tract infection and still has the cough. His past medical history includes asthma for which he takes *Clenil*® 100 mcg 1 puff BD and salbutamol 100 mcg inhale 1–2 puffs QDS PRN. His peak flow is 50% from his best and he is struggling to complete full sentences.
How do you manage Master AB?

- ☐ **A** Offer salbutamol 2.5 mg nebules via inhalation
- ☐ **B** Prescribe amoxicillin and prednisolone for a 5-day course
- ☐ **C** Prescribe oral prednisolone for a 5-day course
- ☐ **D** Prescribe oral prednisolone for a 7-day course
- ☐ **E** Refer to A & E

48 Miss TG, aged 22, presents to the community pharmacy complaining of vaginal itchiness and white creamy discharge. She explains that she recently had a course of antibiotics and has now developed these

symptoms. She has previously had a similar encounter 1 year ago in which she was managed with a fluconazole 50 mg capsule. Upon reviewing the patient and her symptoms, you decide she has vaginal candidiasis.

Which of the following statements is correct regarding fluconazole 50 mg?

- ☐ A   Can be supplied if patient is breastfeeding
- ☐ B   Can be supplied if patient is pregnant
- ☐ C   Can be supplied if patient or partner has been exposed to a sexually transmitted disease
- ☐ D   Can be supplied OTC for patients between the ages of 16–65
- ☐ E   Refer to GP if there have been more than two cases of vaginal candidiasis in the last 6 months

49 Mrs SK, aged 32, presents to the community pharmacy with her 22-month-old son as he is complaining of constipation. She explains they have recently moved to a new house and his diet has lacked fibre in comparison to the last week. He has not opened his bowel for the last 24 hours which is out of the norm for him.

Which of the following is the most appropriate course of action?

- ☐ A   Offer bisacodyl 10 mg suppositories
- ☐ B   Offer lactulose
- ☐ C   Offer senna liquid
- ☐ D   Refer to A & E
- ☐ E   Refer to GP

50 Miss LF, aged 23, presents to the community pharmacy requesting to speak to the pharmacist. She is seeking advice about emergency hormonal contraception. She informs you she has had unprotected sex 12 hours ago and is keen to try the most effective method. Her BMI is 26 kg/m² and she does not take any regular medication for any medical conditions.

Which of the following is the most appropriate course of action?

- ☐ A   Offer *ellaOne*®
- ☐ B   Offer *Levonelle*®
- ☐ C   Refer to A & E
- ☐ D   Refer to GP
- ☐ E   Refer to relevant clinic for insertion of a copper intrauterine device

SECTION B

Oksana Pyzik

1 Mr HS is abroad and presents with symptoms of nausea, abdominal cramps and frequent loose, watery stools.
   Which of the following pathogens is most likely to be implicated in the case of travellers' diarrhoea?

   ☐ A *Borrelia burgdorferi*
   ☐ B *Clostridium botulinum*
   ☐ C *Clostridium difficile*
   ☐ D *Escherichia coli*
   ☐ E *Listeria monocytogenes*

2 Which of the following factors is LEAST likely to increase the risk of contracting travellers' diarrhoea?

   ☐ A Age <6 years
   ☐ B Blood group O
   ☐ C Gender
   ☐ D Use of H_2 receptor antagonists
   ☐ E Use of proton pump inhibitors

3 Which of the following medicines requires monitoring due to dyslipidaemia?

   ☐ A Acamprosate calcium
   ☐ B Alprostadil
   ☐ C Isotretinoin
   ☐ D Moxifloxacin
   ☐ E Ramipril

4 A 27-year-old male has registered to donate blood. Following a medication review he is told that he does not qualify for donation.
   Taking which of the following medicines would mean that this patient must NOT donate blood?

   ☐ A Alitretinoin
   ☐ B Allopurinol
   ☐ C Atenolol
   ☐ D Cyclizine
   ☐ E Salbutamol

5   A father presents at the pharmacy with a prescription for amoxicillin for his 8-year-old child who has been diagnosed with otitis media. The prescription was ordered by the GP three days earlier and the child's symptoms have remained the same over the past three days.
    As the pharmacist, which of the following actions will you take?

   ☐ A   Contact the prescriber and then dispense the medication
   ☐ B   Dispense the medication
   ☐ C   Explain that, at this late date, antibiotic therapy will likely be ineffective for the child
   ☐ D   Refuse to dispense the medication as antibiotics are not recommended
   ☐ E   Refuse to dispense the medication because the prescription is not current

6   Which of the following best describes the term 'cost utility analysis' in the context of a pharmacoeconomic study?

   ☐ A   Is a measurement of the benefit foregone when selecting one therapeutic alternative over the next best alternative
   ☐ B   Is a method for assessing the economic efficiency of proposed public policies through the systematic prediction of social costs and social benefits
   ☐ C   Is an analytical technique intended for the systematic comparative evaluation of the overall cost and benefit generated by alternative therapeutic interventions for the management of a disease
   ☐ D   Is an economic analysis comparing the cost of two similar interventions based on cost
   ☐ E   Is an economic analysis in which the incremental cost of a program from a particular point of view is compared to the incremental health improvement expressed in the unit of quality adjusted life years (QALYs)

Questions 7–9 relate to a 68-year-old man with a history of gout, chronic kidney disease (eGFR = 39 mL/min/1.73m^2) and high cholesterol for which he is currently taking simvastatin 40 mg daily. He has another gout flare up and receives a prescription for naproxen 500 mg BD for 5 days.

7   Which of the following pharmaceutical issues will you flag as the pharmacist?

   ☐ A   Indomethacin should be used for the treatment of acute gout
   ☐ B   Naproxen should be avoided in patients taking simvastatin

☐ **C** Naproxen should be avoided in patients with renal impairment

☐ **D** The duration of naproxen treatment is too short

☐ **E** The naproxen dose is too low

8 The patient was subsequently prescribed allopurinol following successful treatment of the acute attack of gout.
Which of the following counselling points for allopurinol is most appropriate?

☐ **A** Avoid dairy products or multivitamins within 2 hours of dose

☐ **B** Avoid sunlight

☐ **C** Limit fluid intake

☐ **D** Report any skin rash or itching

☐ **E** Take before food

9 The patient asks you what else they can do to prevent further gout attacks in addition to taking the prophylactic medication.
Which one of the following foods should the patient AVOID?

☐ **A** Citrus

☐ **B** Dairy

☐ **C** Eggs

☐ **D** Legumes

☐ **E** Offal

10 Which of the following adverse effects is a patient with a solid cancerous tumour most likely to experience after 1–2 weeks after chemotherapy treatment?

☐ **A** Cardiotoxicity

☐ **B** Emesis

☐ **C** Nephrotoxicity

☐ **D** Neutropenia

☐ **E** Ototoxicity

11 A 78-year-old male with a recent history of urinary tract infection was treated with ciprofloxacin and subsequently developed *Clostridium difficile*-associated diarrhoea (CDAD). He is admitted to hospital with profound diarrhoea, acutely increased serum creatinine concentration and fever (39.5°C).
Based on his symptoms, which of the following is the most appropriate therapy choice?

☐ A   Intravenous metronidazole
☐ B   Intravenous vancomycin
☐ C   Oral cholestyramine
☐ D   Oral metronidazole
☐ E   Oral vancomycin

12 A consultant has asked you to review a new drug to treat diabetes. You review information available on this new drug that is based on a 4-month, placebo-controlled, randomised study of 1000 adults that showed a statistically significant average decrease in Hb1AC from 52 mmol/L to 47 mmol/L. The most common adverse reactions were gastrointestinal symptoms such as abdominal cramping and diarrhoea. Which of the following is the most significant limitation of this study?

☐ A   Hb1AC is a surrogate outcome
☐ B   Long-term safety and efficacy were not assessed
☐ C   Placebo is not an appropriate comparator
☐ D   The patients did not achieve guideline targets for diabetes
☐ E   The sample population was too small to assess efficacy

13 Which of the following best describes a type II error in a study comparing two different medicines as an intervention?

☐ A   The exclusion criteria are not restrictive enough
☐ B   The exclusion criteria are too restrictive
☐ C   The p level is >0.05
☐ D   The statistical conclusion is a false negative stating that there is no difference between the two treatment regimens when there is in fact a difference
☐ E   The statistical conclusion is that there is a difference between the two treatments when it does not actually exist

14 A randomised, controlled trial conducted over 3 years demonstrated that a serious cardiovascular event (primary outcome) occurred in 12% of the patients who received the new drug, whereas the primary outcome occurred in 20% of the patients who received a placebo. What is the relative risk reduction achieved with the new drug?

☐ A   10%
☐ B   15%
☐ C   25%
☐ D   40%
☐ E   50%

15 A 16-year-old female suffers from depression and anxiety. She wants to try cognitive behavioural therapy before starting on antidepressants recommended by the GP. Her parents are very concerned for her wellbeing as her marks have suffered in the last year and pressure the GP to prescribe medication.

From an ethics perspective, which principle is being violated?

- ☐ A   Autonomy
- ☐ B   Confidentiality
- ☐ C   Justice
- ☐ D   Nonmaleficence
- ☐ E   Veracity

16 Which of the following medicines is safe to take during pregnancy?

- ☐ A   Ibuprofen
- ☐ B   Insulin
- ☐ C   Isotretinoin
- ☐ D   Metformin
- ☐ E   Propranolol

17 A 69-year-old female is diagnosed with hypothyroidism and is initiated on low dose levothyroxine. She weighs 65 kg and has a history of diabetes and osteoporosis and is taking metformin and alendronic acid. Which of the following is the most likely rationale for the low dose of levothyroxine?

- ☐ A   Age
- ☐ B   Diabetic
- ☐ C   Drug interaction
- ☐ D   Gender
- ☐ E   Weight

18 Which one of the following is LEAST likely to cause acute pancreatitis?

- ☐ A   Alcohol
- ☐ B   Azathioprine
- ☐ C   Gallstones
- ☐ D   Propranolol
- ☐ E   Trimethoprim-sulfamethoxazole

19 A 61-year-old male has been admitted to hospital after suffering a minor stroke. He has a history of type 2 diabetes, DVT, hypertension and hypercholesterolaemia.

Which of the following medicines should be DISCONTINUED?

- ☐ **A**   Bendroflumethiazide
- ☐ **B**   Bezafibrate
- ☐ **C**   Enoxaparin
- ☐ **D**   Metformin
- ☐ **E**   Simvastatin

20 Anaphylactic shock is associated with airway oedema.
Which of the following is the most appropriate treatment in the first instance?

- ☐ **A**   Adrenaline
- ☐ **B**   IV chlorphenamine
- ☐ **C**   IV hydrocortisone
- ☐ **D**   Oxygen
- ☐ **E**   Salbutamol

21 Which one of the following is the most appropriate product to treat a case of diagnosed corneal oedema?

- ☐ **A**   Antihistamine
- ☐ **B**   Artificial tears
- ☐ **C**   Hyperosmotic agent
- ☐ **D**   Vasoconstrictor
- ☐ **E**   Vasodilator

22 A 64-year-old male has a history of angina and is starting to develop signs of tolerance.
Which of the following statements is correct regarding nitrate tolerance?

- ☐ **A**   Tolerance does not occur with sublingual glyceryl trinitrate
- ☐ **B**   Tolerance does not occur with transdermal nitroglycerin
- ☐ **C**   Tolerance is dependent on age of patient
- ☐ **D**   Tolerance is dependent on route of administration
- ☐ **E**   Tolerance may be prevented by intermittent nitrate administration

23 A 35-year-old male is admitted into hospital with ulcerative colitis. He is dehydrated due to diarrhoea with more than eight stools per day with fresh blood. There is no evidence of obstruction and blood tests show inflammatory markers are within the target range.

Which of the following treatment options is most appropriate for this patient?

- [ ] **A**   Administer IV hydrocortisone 100 mg QDS
- [ ] **B**   Administer 1L 5% IV dextrose over 24 hours
- [ ] **C**   Administer mesalazine suppository
- [ ] **D**   Administer two loperamide capsules straight away and after each loose stool
- [ ] **E**   Administer IV metronidazole 500 mg TDS

24 Which of the following antineoplastic treatments is DNA-binding?

- [ ] **A**   Docetaxel
- [ ] **B**   Doxorubicin
- [ ] **C**   Trabectedin
- [ ] **D**   Vinblastine
- [ ] **E**   Vincristine

25 Which of the following cancer treatments is NOT a type of immunotherapy?

- [ ] **A**   Degarelix (*Firmagon*®)
- [ ] **B**   Interferon
- [ ] **C**   Ipilimumab (*Yervoy*®)
- [ ] **D**   Nivolumab (*Opdivo*®)
- [ ] **E**   Tisagenlecleucel (*Kymirah*®)

26 Which of the following best describes the frequency of rarely reported side effects?

- [ ] **A** $\geq 1/100$ to $<1/10$
- [ ] **B** $\geq 1/1000$ to $<1/100$
- [ ] **C** $\geq 1/10,000$ to $<1/100$
- [ ] **D** $\geq 1/100,000$ to $<1/10,000$
- [ ] **E** $<1/100,000,000$

27 A 21-year-old female complains of frequent nightmares.
Which one of the following medicines is LEAST likely to be linked to these side effects?

- [ ] **A**   Buspirone
- [ ] **B**   Paroxetine
- [ ] **C**   Propranolol
- [ ] **D**   Sertraline
- [ ] **E**   Zopiclone

28 A 75-year-old female with a history of osteoarthritis, hypertension, and anaemia is hospitalised due to severe oedema, shortness of breath and decreased urine output. Her blood tests results are as follows:

	Value
Potassium	5.1 mmol/L
Urea	12 mmol/L
Creatinine	240 μmol/L

Which of the following medicines would you recommend that the prescriber STOP immediately?

- ☐ A   Alendronic acid 70 mg once weekly
- ☐ B   Calcium carbonate 1500 mg and vitamin D3 (400 IU) OD
- ☐ C   Ferrous sulfate 200 mg TDS
- ☐ D   Propranolol 40 mg BD
- ☐ E   Ramipril 5 mg OD

29 A 54-year-female is admitted into hospital after presenting with convulsions, visual disturbances, confusion and a visible coarse tremor. The patient is taking lithium, tibolone and has recently been prescribed bendroflumethiazide. On admission, tests for urine and electrolytes were performed.
Which of the following electrolyte values would you expect to be ABNORMAL?

- ☐ A   Calcium
- ☐ B   Creatinine
- ☐ C   Potassium
- ☐ D   Sodium
- ☐ E   Urea

30 Which of the following statements is correct regarding virus vectors used in the production of biotechnology drugs?

- ☐ A   Rotavirus is a poor viral vector for gene therapy
- ☐ B   The most frequent source of virus introduction is the growth media
- ☐ C   Viruses can be generated by an infected production cell line
- ☐ D   Viruses cannot be inactivated by physical treatment of the product
- ☐ E   Viruses cannot be introduced by nutrients

31 Which of the following is the correct route of administration for vincristine?

    ☐ **A**   Intrathecal
    ☐ **B**   Intravenous
    ☐ **C**   Oral
    ☐ **D**   Rectal
    ☐ **E**   Subcutaneous

32 A 63-year-old man with type 2 diabetes, congestive heart failure and ischaemic left ventricular dysfunction presented with chest discomfort. Physical examination revealed severe gynaecomastia.
Which of his following medicines is most likely to have induced gynaecomastia?

    ☐ **A**   Amlodipine
    ☐ **B**   Bisoprolol
    ☐ **C**   Metformin
    ☐ **D**   Ramipril
    ☐ **E**   Spironolactone

33 A 19-year-old female presents at the pharmacy with symptoms of dysuria, lower abdominal pain, vaginal discharge and bleeding between menstrual cycles and heavy bleeding after intercourse. She has no previous history of abnormal menstrual cycles.
Which of the following conditions is the most likely diagnosis for this patient?

    ☐ **A**   Chlamydia
    ☐ **B**   Oligomenorrhea
    ☐ **C**   Primary dysmenorrhoea
    ☐ **D**   Secondary amenorrhoea
    ☐ **E**   Trichomonas vaginalis

34 Which of the following is the correct blood volume of an average adult?

    ☐ **A**   3 L
    ☐ **B**   5 L
    ☐ **C**   8 L
    ☐ **D**   12 L
    ☐ **E**   24 L

35 Which of the following factors is the most appropriate determinant of bioequivalence between two different brands of medicines?

☐ A Package size
☐ B Pharmacokinetic parameters
☐ C Price of medicine
☐ D Tablet size
☐ E Taste of medicine

36 Which of the following pathogens is most likely to cause community-acquired pneumonia in adults?

☐ A *Chlamydophila pneumoniae*
☐ B *Haemophilus influenzae*
☐ C *Parainfluenza virus*
☐ D *Pneumocystis jirovecii*
☐ E *Streptococcus pneumoniae*

Questions 37–39 relate to a 19-year-old-female who presents with symptoms of hirsutism, hair loss from the head and acne. She has recently had an ultrasound which revealed an increased ovarian volume and twelve peripheral follicles.

37 Which of the following is the most likely condition that this patient is suffering from?

☐ A Cervical dysplasia
☐ B Cushing's syndrome
☐ C Endometriosis
☐ D Hypothyroidism
☐ E Polycystic ovary syndrome

38 Which of the following medicines is most appropriate to treat this patient's condition?

☐ A Ibuprofen
☐ B Levothyroxine
☐ C Metformin
☐ D Metyrapone
☐ E Naproxen

39 Which of the following is LEAST likely to be linked to the patient's condition?

☐ A Cervical cancer
☐ B Diabetes
☐ C Infertility
☐ D Insulin resistance
☐ E Obesity

40 A 38-year-old female is 26 weeks pregnant and is admitted into hospital
with severe hypertension (160/110 mmHg) and proteinuria. She has had
an increasing number of severe headaches throughout her pregnancy
which is relieved by regular analgesics and presents with oedema of the
hands and feet.
Which one of the following is the most likely diagnosis?

    □ **A**   Ectopic pregnancy
    □ **B**   Gestational diabetes
    □ **C**   Hyperemesis gravidarum
    □ **D**   Placenta previa
    □ **E**   Pre-eclampsia

41 A 50-year-old male who suffers from depression has recently suffered a
myocardial infarction and is switched to another antidepressant.
Which of the following antidepressants is most appropriate for this
patient?

    □ **A**   Bupropion
    □ **B**   Citalopram
    □ **C**   Doxepin
    □ **D**   Sertraline
    □ **E**   Venlafaxine

42 A 50-year-old male presents at your pharmacy complaining of stomach
pains and nausea which has gradually become worse over the past
3–4 days. He describes his pain as gnawing and generalised over his
abdomen and is most painful at night. Over the past 24 hours he passed
several loose stools that he described as dark, tarry and foul smelling
but had not seen frank diarrhoea or fresh blood. He is taking the
following medication: atenolol 50 mg OD, diclofenac 50 mg TDS.
Which of the following is the most likely diagnosis?

    □ **A**   Acid reflux
    □ **B**   Duodenal ulcer
    □ **C**   Gastric cancer
    □ **D**   Indigestion
    □ **E**   Stomach ulcer

43 The most common cause of sciatica is a herniated intervertebral disc.
Which of the following vertebrae is most frequently affected?

    □ **A**   L1
    □ **B**   L1-L2
    □ **C**   L2-L3

☐ **D** L4-L5
☐ **E** L5

44 Orlistat is contraindicated in patients with which of the following condition?

☐ **A** Asthma
☐ **B** Cholestasis
☐ **C** Diabetes
☐ **D** Emphysema
☐ **E** Glaucoma

45 A 6-year-old boy presents with throbbing pain in the left ear with mucopurulent discharge. He has no other symptoms.
Which one of the following treatments would be most appropriate for this patient?

☐ **A** Acetic acid
☐ **B** Amoxicillin
☐ **C** Hydrocortisone
☐ **D** Hydrogen peroxide
☐ **E** Paracetamol

46 A 16-year-old male with a suspected case of strep throat was prescribed antibiotics for his sore throat, but following treatment his symptoms have not subsided and he also develops fever, swollen lymph nodes, headache, skin rash and severe fatigue. You begin to suspect that the patient was misdiagnosed and that he may be suffering from infectious mononucleosis.
Which of the following pathogens causes mononucleosis?

☐ **A** *Epstein-Barr virus*
☐ **B** *Norovirus*
☐ **C** *Parainfluenza virus*
☐ **D** *Paramyxovirus*
☐ **E** *Parvovirus B19*

47 A 35-year-old female presents at the pharmacy requesting a topical treatment for her face as she has a patch of papules and pustules across her cheeks and chin, generalised dry skin and broken capillaries across her forehead and cheeks. The redness is most prominent around her cheeks and appears flushed.

Which of the following medicines is the most appropriate first-line treatment for this patient?

- ☐ A Adapalene
- ☐ B Azelaic acid
- ☐ C Co-pyrindiol
- ☐ D Emollient
- ☐ E Metronidazole

48 How many fingertip units of hydrocortisone are required to cover the entire leg and foot of a 4-year-old child?

- ☐ A 1.5 units
- ☐ B 2 units
- ☐ C 3 units
- ☐ D 3.5 units
- ☐ E 4 units

49 An 89-year-old male presents with cracking at the corners of the lips which he describes as a burning pain. His mouth is also dry at the corners. He wears dentures and frequently licks his lips.
Which of the following is the most likely diagnosis?

- ☐ A Allergic dermatitis
- ☐ B Angular cheilitis
- ☐ C Cold sore
- ☐ D Impetigo
- ☐ E Molluscum contagiosum

50 Which of the following risk factors is LEAST likely to be associated with peptic ulcers?

- ☐ A Age
- ☐ B Antibiotics
- ☐ C Blood type
- ☐ D *H. pylori*
- ☐ E NSAIDs

SECTION C

Pratik Thakkar

1 A patient has been recently prescribed simvastatin. You are counselling the patient on this medicine and what to look out for.
  Which of the following fruit juices should be AVOIDED when taking a statin?

  - ☐ A Apple juice
  - ☐ B Grapefruit juice
  - ☐ C Mixed berry juice
  - ☐ D Orange juice
  - ☐ E Pineapple juice

2 A 60-year-old patient with COPD is on the following regular medications: aspirin 75 mg OD, ramipril 5 mg OD, tiotropium inhaler 18 mg OD, simvastatin 40 mg ON and bisoprolol 2.5 mg OD. His GP has started him on a course of clarithromycin for an infective exacerbation of his COPD.
  Which of his regular medications should be WITHELD whilst taking clarithromycin?

  - ☐ A Aspirin
  - ☐ B Bisoprolol
  - ☐ C Ramipril
  - ☐ D Simvastatin
  - ☐ E Tiotropium

Questions 3–5 relate to the same patient.

3 A 41-year-old woman with a history of epilepsy and mental health problems is admitted to A & E with confusion following a seizure earlier in the day. She has also had severe diarrhoea and vomiting. On examination she is noted to have a coarse tremor, her blood pressure is 124/71 mmHg and her heart rate is 64 bpm. She is dehydrated and her body temperature is 36.7°C.
  What is the most likely diagnosis?

  - ☐ A Lithium toxicity
  - ☐ B Neuroleptic malignant syndrome
  - ☐ C Serotonin withdrawal syndrome
  - ☐ D Sodium valproate overdose
  - ☐ E Tricyclic overdose

4   She had recently been commenced on an antihypertensive medication by her GP as her ambulatory blood pressure readings showed an average BP of 150/90 mmHg. She is on the following medications already – sodium valproate, lithium and levothyroxine.
   Which of the following antihypertensives is safest to commence in her case?

   ☐ A   Amlodipine
   ☐ B   Bendroflumethiazide
   ☐ C   Furosemide
   ☐ D   Losartan
   ☐ E   Ramipril

5   Her initial blood work returns from the lab. Her blood test results are as follows:

	Value	Normal range
Lithium	2.5 mmol/L	0.4–1.0 mmol/L
Serum sodium	150 mmol/L	135–145 mmol/L
Serum potassium	5.2 mmol/L	3.5–5.2 mmol/L
Urea	7.4 mmol/L	2.5–7.0 mmol/L
Creatinine	152 μmol/L	45–90 μmol/L
eGFR	43 mL/min/1.73 m^2	>90 mL/min/1.73 m^2

   What is the most appropriate management?

   ☐ A   Haemodialysis
   ☐ B   IV 0.9% normal saline
   ☐ C   IV 5% dextrose
   ☐ D   IV Hartmann's solution
   ☐ E   IV sodium bicarbonate

6   A patient has been on chemotherapy for lung cancer. He has rising levels of uric acid. The doctors have prescribed allopurinol as adjunct treatment to avoid hyperuricaemia.
   What is the mechanism of action of allopurinol?

   ☐ A   Angiotensin converting enzyme inhibitor
   ☐ B   HMG-CoA reductase inhibitor
   ☐ C   Monoamine oxidase inhibitor
   ☐ D   Phosphodiesterase-5 inhibitor
   ☐ E   Xanthine oxidase inhibitor

7   A 45-year-old man presents to the community pharmacist complaining of a 2-day history of fever and sore throat. He is normally fit and well and his only regular medication is carbimazole for hyperthyroidism, which was commenced 2 months ago.
Which of the following is the most suitable recommended action?

☐ **A**   Advise him to see his GP to get antibiotics
☐ **B**   Advise him to watch and wait
☐ **C**   Recommend difflam spray
☐ **D**   Tell him to go to A & E for blood tests
☐ **E**   Tell him to take PRN paracetamol at home

8   A 52-year-old gentleman has just been started on azathioprine for Crohn's disease.
Which of the following of his regular repeat medications should be STOPPED?

☐ **A**   Allopurinol
☐ **B**   Amlodipine
☐ **C**   Atorvastatin
☐ **D**   Mebeverine
☐ **E**   Omeprazole

9   Which of the following criteria is NOT part of the CURB-65 score in the assessment of community-acquired pneumonia?

☐ **A**   Age of the patient
☐ **B**   Blood pressure
☐ **C**   C-reactive protein level
☐ **D**   Respiratory rate
☐ **E**   Urea level

10   A 64-year-old lady with Addison's disease is admitted to hospital with pyelonephritis and is started on IV antibiotics. She is normally on 20 mg hydrocortisone OM and 10 mg hydrocortisone ON.
What should happen to her steroid dosing whilst acutely unwell in hospital?

☐ **A**   No change to dosing
☐ **B**   Switch to an equivalent dose of fludrocortisone
☐ **C**   Take 10 mg OM and 5 mg ON
☐ **D**   Take 20 mg BD
☐ **E**   Take 40 mg OM and 20 mg ON

11   A 23-year-old gentleman who has recently moved to the UK from Bangladesh has been diagnosed with tuberculosis.

Which of the following drugs can cause his bodily secretions to turn a reddish/brown colour?

- ☐ **A**   Ethambutol
- ☐ **B**   Isoniazid
- ☐ **C**   Pyrazinamide
- ☐ **D**   Pyridoxine
- ☐ **E**   Rifampicin

12 An 18-year-old girl comes to the community pharmacy seeking emergency contraception. She had unprotected sexual intercourse 4 days ago. Her last period was 2 weeks ago.
What is the most recommended form of contraception to give her, assuming there are no contraindications?

- ☐ **A**   1.5 mg levonorgestrel
- ☐ **B**   30 mg ulipristal acetate
- ☐ **C**   Copper IUD
- ☐ **D**   Depot progestogen injections
- ☐ **E**   Mirena coil

13 A 30-year-old woman presents to A & E with palpitations. An ECG taken shows that she is in supraventricular tachycardia with a heart rate of 130 bpm. She is haemodynamically stable with a BP reading of 123/80 mmHg.
What is the most appropriate first-line treatment for her arrhythmia?

- ☐ **A**   Adenosine
- ☐ **B**   Bisoprolol
- ☐ **C**   Flecainide
- ☐ **D**   Valsalva manoeuvre
- ☐ **E**   Verapamil

14 A 19-year-old cocaine addict is admitted to hospital with chest pain. On examination he is found to be hypertensive with a BP reading of 180/100 mmHg and tachycardic with a heart rate of 104 bpm.
Which of the following symptoms would you expect to see in this patient?

- ☐ **A**   Hyperkalaemia
- ☐ **B**   Hypernatraemia
- ☐ **C**   Hyperthermia
- ☐ **D**   Hypokalaemia
- ☐ **E**   Hypothermia

15 What is the mechanism of action of clopidogrel?

    ☐ **A**   Enhances the effect of circulating antithrombin
    ☐ **B**   Inhibits binding of adenosine diphosphate
    ☐ **C**   Inhibits cyclo-oxygenase-1
    ☐ **D**   Irreversibly binds glycoprotein IIb/IIIa receptor sites
    ☐ **E**   Prevents production of thromboxane A2

16 A 74-year-old gentleman with type 2 diabetes has recently been started on dapagliflozin as part of his diabetic regimen.
What is the most important effect to warn him about with this class of medication?

    ☐ **A**   Can cause headaches
    ☐ **B**   Can cause light headedness
    ☐ **C**   Can cause weight gain
    ☐ **D**   Can increase the risk of urinary tract infections
    ☐ **E**   Hypoglycaemic effects

17 Which of the following groups of people are eligible for the annual intramuscular influenza vaccine free of charge on the NHS?

    ☐ **A**   BMI >35
    ☐ **B**   Children aged between 2 and 17 years
    ☐ **C**   People over the age of 60 years
    ☐ **D**   People with acute kidney injury
    ☐ **E**   People with chronic heart failure

18 A 61-year-old man with metastatic prostate cancer is on oral morphine sulphate 30 mg capsules BD.
What is the maximum dose of liquid oral morphine 10 mg/5 mL solution that can be given to him for breakthrough pain?

    ☐ **A**   5 mg
    ☐ **B**   10 mg
    ☐ **C**   15 mg
    ☐ **D**   20 mg
    ☐ **E**   30 mg

19 A 44-year-old lady is on gabapentin 300 mg TDS for chronic pain, secondary to her fibromyalgia.

What is the maximum recommended duration of supply on a single prescription for this medication?

    ☐ **A**   7 days
    ☐ **B**   28 days
    ☐ **C**   30 days
    ☐ **D**   3 months
    ☐ **E**   6 months

20 A 75-year-old type 2 diabetic was found unconscious at home by his wife. A blue light ambulance was called. On arrival at his house, the paramedics found that his blood sugar was 0.8 mmol/L and he had a Glasgow Coma Scale score of 3.
Which of the following is the quickest way to raise his blood sugar safely?

    ☐ **A**   Establish IV access and put up IV 5% dextrose drip
    ☐ **B**   Establish IV access and put up IV 50% dextrose drip
    ☐ **C**   IM glucagon
    ☐ **D**   IM insulin
    ☐ **E**   Oral lucozade

21 Which of the following medicines when used in isolation is most likely to induce hypoglycaemia?

    ☐ **A**   Gliclazide
    ☐ **B**   Metformin
    ☐ **C**   Nateglinide
    ☐ **D**   Pioglitazone
    ☐ **E**   Sitagliptin

22 A 45-year-old Afro-Caribbean man has been diagnosed with essential hypertension. His BP is 157/98 mmHg. He needs to start on antihypertensive medication. He does not have any other medical conditions and has no known allergies.
Which of the following medications is the most appropriate to commence?

    ☐ **A**   Amlodipine
    ☐ **B**   Bendroflumethiazide
    ☐ **C**   Bisoprolol
    ☐ **D**   Losartan
    ☐ **E**   Ramipril

23 An 11-year-old child has had a longstanding diagnosis of asthma for which she takes a salbutamol inhaler PRN. More recently, she had started to experience a dry nocturnal cough that is keeping her up at least three times a week.
Which of the following medications should be started in addition to her salbutamol?

☐ **A** Aminophylline
☐ **B** Beclometasone dipropionate
☐ **C** Montelukast
☐ **D** Oral prednisolone
☐ **E** Salmeterol

24 A 37-year-old woman with a history of depression was brought to hospital having been found unconscious at home. She had written a suicide note and had an empty bottle of amitriptyline in her jacket.
What is the most appropriate initial intravenous treatment?

☐ **A** 0.9% sodium chloride
☐ **B** Dextrose
☐ **C** Hartmann's solution
☐ **D** Magnesium
☐ **E** Sodium bicarbonate

25 An 18-year-old student was brought to A & E after collapsing at a night club. On arrival, her respiratory rate was 12, Glasgow Coma Scale was reduced at 10 and her pupils were pinpoint in both eyes.
Which of the following drugs is she most likely to have abused?

☐ **A** Cocaine
☐ **B** Ecstasy
☐ **C** Heroin
☐ **D** MDMA
☐ **E** Methanol

26 An 83-year-old woman who is normally fit and well has been complaining of an irresistible urge to move her legs at night which she is finding increasingly distressing. Her GP has diagnosed her with restless leg syndrome.
Which of the following medications is the most appropriate to give her to ameliorate her symptoms?

☐ **A** Co-careldopa
☐ **B** Diazepam

- [ ] **C**   Pramipexole
- [ ] **D**   Propranolol
- [ ] **E**   Quinine sulphate

27   A 25-year-old pregnant lady comes to see you as she is concerned that she had come into contact with her 3-year-old niece on the day she developed chickenpox. Her booking bloods at pregnancy show that she has not had chickenpox previously herself.
What is the recommended course of action?

- [ ] **A**   Advise her that it is too late and nothing can be done
- [ ] **B**   Give her the varicella vaccination
- [ ] **C**   Give her varicella immunoglobulin
- [ ] **D**   Treat with oral aciclovir
- [ ] **E**   Watch and wait, and treat only if she develops chicken pox

28   A 75-year-old gentleman goes to his local community pharmacist wishing to purchase sildenafil. He has a background of ischaemic heart disease and hypertension.
Which of the following medications would mean he should NOT take the sildenafil?

- [ ] **A**   Amlodipine
- [ ] **B**   Aspirin
- [ ] **C**   Bendroflumethiazide
- [ ] **D**   Isosorbide mononitrate
- [ ] **E**   Ramipril

Questions 29 and 30 relate to the same patient.

29   An 80-year-old female patient is admitted to the hospital as she has been feeling generally unwell and has been unable to eat or drink for the past 24 hours. She has a background of chronic low back pain for which she is on regular oral morphine sulphate. Whilst in hospital she is found to be increasingly drowsy with reduced respiratory rate and pinpoint pupils. A diagnosis of opioid toxicity is made.
What is the most likely cause of this?

- [ ] **A**   Acute liver failure
- [ ] **B**   Acute renal failure
- [ ] **C**   Acute respiratory distress syndrome
- [ ] **D**   Delirium
- [ ] **E**   Sepsis

30 Which of the following should be administered to help alleviate her symptoms of opioid toxicity?

    □ **A**   Flumazenil
    □ **B**   IV antibiotics
    □ **C**   Naloxone
    □ **D**   Nebulised salbutamol
    □ **E**   Nebulised saline

Questions 31–33 relate to the same patient.

31 An 18-year-old girl wishes to start an oral contraceptive pill before starting university. She has regular periods and is not on any regular medications.
Which of the following would be an absolute contraindication to the prescription of the combined oral contraceptive pill?

    □ **A**   BMI of 32
    □ **B**   Family history of breast cancer
    □ **C**   First degree relative with DVT at 44 years
    □ **D**   Migraine with aura
    □ **E**   Smoker of five cigarettes per day

32 Given the above absolute contraindication to the prescription of the combined oral contraceptive pill, her GP has given her a prescription for the progestogen-only pill.
Which of the following side effects is more common with the progestogen-only pill when compared to the combined pill?

    □ **A**   Improvement of acne
    □ **B**   Irregular periods
    □ **C**   Migraine
    □ **D**   Venous thromboembolism
    □ **E**   Weight gain

33 She would prefer to take a progestogen-only pill with a longer window period in case of a missed pill.
Which of the following progestogen-only pills has a 12-hour window?

    □ **A**   *Cerazette*® (desogestrel)
    □ **B**   *Femulen*® (etynodiol)
    □ **C**   *Micronor*® (norethisterone)
    □ **D**   *Norgeston*® (levonorgestrel)
    □ **E**   *Noriday*® (norethisterone)

Questions 34–36 relate to the same patient.

34 A patient presents to A & E following a deliberate overdose of 50 × 500 mg paracetamol tablets 4 hours ago. Initial bloods show raised paracetamol levels which requires treatment.
What is the drug of choice to give her?

☐ **A** Activated charcoal
☐ **B** Glucagon
☐ **C** Methanol
☐ **D** N-acetylcysteine
☐ **E** Sodium bicarbonate

35 What is the mechanism of action of N-acetylcysteine?

☐ **A** Binds toxic metabolites
☐ **B** Promotes breakdown of toxic metabolites
☐ **C** Promotes renal excretion of paracetamol
☐ **D** Reduces glutathione levels
☐ **E** Replenishes glutathione levels

36 Which of these is the preferred choice of treatment for paracetamol overdose more than 8 hours after ingestion of the toxic dose?

☐ **A** Activated charcoal
☐ **B** Gastric lavage
☐ **C** Haemodialysis
☐ **D** Hepatic transplant
☐ **E** N-acetylcysteine administration

37 A 25-year-old female has a persistent fungal nail infection despite 6 months treatment with topical amlorifine. Her GP has sent nail clippings for a fungal culture which has come back positive for tinea pedis.
Which of the following is the next best management option?

☐ **A** Oral fluconazole
☐ **B** Oral miconazole
☐ **C** Oral nystatin
☐ **D** Oral terbinafine
☐ **E** Topical nystatin

Questions 38–40 relate to the same patient.

38 A 52-year-old businessman who drinks four pints of beer each night has recently been started on naproxen for an acute tendon injury by his GP following an injury sustained to his shoulder whilst abroad. He has a past medical history of depression for which he is on sertraline. He has

also had a cholecystectomy for gallstone disease in the past. He presents to the GP two weeks later with severe epigastric pain and a history of vomiting, including noticing some fresh red blood in his vomit.
What is the most likely cause of his abdominal pain?

- ☐ A Acute pancreatitis
- ☐ B Appendicitis
- ☐ C Diverticulitis
- ☐ D Gastroenteritis
- ☐ E Peptic ulcer

39 The patient has been seen by the gastric team and they record that there is a confirmed gastric bleed.
What is the most likely cause of this?

- ☐ A Eating too many fatty foods
- ☐ B Gallstone disease
- ☐ C Interaction between naproxen and sertraline
- ☐ D Recent travel abroad
- ☐ E Reheating his takeaway from three nights ago

40 What preventive measure could have been taken to AVOID this condition?

- ☐ A Advise him to continue on his current diet
- ☐ B Advise him to stop drinking whilst on naproxen
- ☐ C Co-prescribe a PPI with naproxen
- ☐ D Stop sertraline while on naproxen
- ☐ E Tell him to take aspirin instead of naproxen

41 A 45-year-old gentleman has recently attended the smoking cessation clinic. He has a past history of epilepsy and depression for which he takes lamotrigine and sertraline.
Which of the following medications should be AVOIDED in his case?

- ☐ A Bupropion
- ☐ B Nicotine gum
- ☐ C Nicotine inhalator
- ☐ D Nicotine patch
- ☐ E Varenicline

42 A 34-year-old man with a past history of HIV infection presents to the emergency department with watery diarrhoea. He is currently on HIV treatment. The viral load is undetectable and CD4 count is

800 and therefore not severely immunocompromised. *Cryptosporidium* infection is confirmed on ZN (Ziehl-Neelsen) staining.
What is the most suitable management?

- ☐ A   Amoxicillin
- ☐ B   Ciprofloxacin
- ☐ C   Co-trimoxazole
- ☐ D   Metronidazole
- ☐ E   Supportive therapy

Questions 43–46 relate to the same patient.

43   A 15-year-old girl is under the care of the dermatologist for severe acne vulgaris. She is currently being treated with once daily oral lymecycline. What is the most important side effect to warn her about?

- ☐ A   Blue discolouration of vision
- ☐ B   Discoloration of urine
- ☐ C   Photosensitivity
- ☐ D   Tendinopathy
- ☐ E   Tingling of peripheries

44   She returns for review 3 months later. Unfortunately, there has been no response to treatment and examination reveals evidence of widespread scarring on her face. What is the next most suitable treatment?

- ☐ A   IV retinoids
- ☐ B   Oral retinoids
- ☐ C   Topical antibiotics and benzoyl peroxide
- ☐ D   Topical retinoids
- ☐ E   Trial of oral doxycycline

45   You receive a prescription for isotretinoin, and you are counselling the patient on common side effects.
What is the most common side effect to warn the patient about that majority of other patients will experience?

- ☐ A   Anxiety
- ☐ B   Dryness of skin and lips
- ☐ C   Hyperhidrosis
- ☐ D   Nail dystrophy
- ☐ E   Photosensitivity reaction

46 What should be checked each time a new prescription of a retinoid is signed for by the doctor?

    ☐ A   Full blood count
    ☐ B   Kidney function
    ☐ C   Liver function
    ☐ D   Pregnancy test
    ☐ E   Thyroid function

47 A 27-year-old lady with a history of generalised tonic-clonic seizures comes to see you following the birth of her first baby. She had an uncomplicated pregnancy and wishes to breastfeed.
Which of the following antiepileptic medications is safe for her to use whilst breastfeeding?

    ☐ A   Lamotrigine
    ☐ B   Phenytoin
    ☐ C   Sodium valproate
    ☐ D   All the above
    ☐ E   None of the above

48 An 8-week-old baby has just been seen by the GP at the 6–8-week baby check and has been noted to have moderate 'cradle cap'. The parents have been advised to see the pharmacist to suggest the best treatment for this condition.
Which of the following is the first line of treatment?

    ☐ A   1% hydrocortisone cream
    ☐ B   Baby shampoo and baby oil
    ☐ C   Refer back to GP as they should be referred to a dermatologist
    ☐ D   Topical ketoconazole shampoo
    ☐ E   Watch and wait

Questions 49 and 50 relate to the same patient.

49 A 7-year-old boy has recently been prescribed permethrin 5% cream. Which condition is this the first-line recommended treatment for?

    ☐ A   Acne vulgaris
    ☐ B   Chicken pox
    ☐ C   Head lice
    ☐ D   Scabies
    ☐ E   Tinea corporis (ringworm)

50 The patient's mother has presented with a prescription of permethrin 5% cream.
How soon after the initial treatment is a second course required?

- □ A   24 hours
- □ B   48 hours
- □ C   1 week
- □ D   2 weeks
- □ E   1 month

51 The General Pharmaceutical Council (GPhC) is the regulator for pharmacists, pharmacy technicians and pharmacy premises.
Which of the following is NOT a principle function of the GPhC?

- □ A   Approving qualifications for pharmacists and pharmacy technicians
- □ B   Maintaining a register of pharmacists, pharmacy technicians and pharmacy premises
- □ C   Promoting pharmacy in the media, government and leading the way in medicines information
- □ D   Setting standards for conduct, ethics, proficiency, education and training, and continuing professional development (CPD)
- □ E   Stablishing fitness to practise requirements, monitoring pharmacy professionals' fitness to practise and dealing firmly and fairly with complaints

52 According to the GPhC Standards for Pharmacy Professionals, which of the following is NOT a criteria for standard 1 – 'Pharmacy professionals must provide person-centred care.'?
Pharmacy professionals should:

- □ A   Consider the impact of their practice whether or not they provide care directly
- □ B   Give the person all relevant information in a way they can understand so they can make informed decisions and choices
- □ C   Involve, support and enable every person when making decisions about their health, care and wellbeing
- □ D   Obtain consent to provide care and pharmacy services
- □ E   Recognise their own values and beliefs and impose them on other people

53 A patient has been admitted to hospital with moderate diarrhoea and a suspected *C. difficile* infection. The patient is allergic to penicillin.

Which antibiotic is appropriate for treatment of their suspected infection-related diarrhoea?

- ☐ A Caspofungin
- ☐ B Co-amoxiclav
- ☐ C Flucloxacillin
- ☐ D Metronidazole
- ☐ E Vancomycin

Questions 54 and 55 are related to a female patient who has been treated with vancomycin in hospital for infective endocarditis. She is 60 years old and weighs 65 kg. You may use the SPC for vancomycin to help you: https://www.medicines.org.uk/emc/product/649/smpc

54 The patient has a creatinine clearance of 45 mL/min.
What is the highest starting dose of vancomycin that can be given?

- ☐ A 975 mg
- ☐ B 1000 mg
- ☐ C 1100 mg
- ☐ D 1200 mg
- ☐ E 1300 mg

55 The nursing team are asking for the most appropriate diluent for the infusion of vancomycin.
Which of the following according to the SPC is a suitable diluent for vancomycin?

- ☐ A Glucose 10% injection
- ☐ B Sodium chloride 0.45% / glucose 2.5%
- ☐ C Sodium chloride 0.45% / glucose 5%
- ☐ D Sodium chloride 9 mg/mL (0.9%) injection
- ☐ E Water for injection

56 Which of the following side effects most commonly occurs due to fast infusion of vancomycin?

- ☐ A Acute tubular necrosis
- ☐ B Diarrhoea
- ☐ C Erythematous rash or 'red man syndrome'
- ☐ D Nausea
- ☐ E Vasculitis

57 An 80-year-old female inpatient with schizophrenia has been on haloperidol long term with no previous issues. She has recently been

prescribed another medication to control her symptoms. She has developed a temperature of 38.6°C and increasing muscle rigidity.
Which is the single most likely cause of her symptoms?

- ☐ **A** Amitriptyline
- ☐ **B** Diazepam
- ☐ **C** Flupentixol
- ☐ **D** Sertraline
- ☐ **E** Zopiclone

58 A 50-year-old Caucasian man visits your practice for a check-up. It is the first time he has visited a GP practice and was encouraged to visit by his wife. He has no significant medical history and he is found to have a blood pressure of 158/90 mmHg. He is not a smoker or diabetic, with no other significant history other than being overweight.
What is the single best initial management?

- ☐ **A** ACE inhibitors
- ☐ **B** Advise lifestyle measures
- ☐ **C** Angiotensin receptor blockers
- ☐ **D** Beta blockers
- ☐ **E** Calcium channel antagonist

59 A 60-year-old man presents to your pharmacy complaining of bilateral knee pain. He likely has osteoarthritis.
What is the most appropriate first-line treatment option for this patient?

- ☐ **A** Amitriptyline
- ☐ **B** Aspirin
- ☐ **C** Celecoxib
- ☐ **D** Ibuprofen
- ☐ **E** Paracetamol

Questions 60 and 61 relate to a patient who presents to your pharmacy with pain in his leg.

60 A 42-year-old man felt a sharp pain at the back of his ankle while playing badminton. He thought that somebody may have kicked him from behind. He is now unable to walk normally. On examination there is no pain when pressing against the calf muscle, tibia and metatarsal area of the heel. There was a sharp pain when pressing against the back of the ankle in a concentrated area only.
What is the most likely diagnosis?

☐ **A**   Achilles tendon rupture
☐ **B**   Ankle fracture
☐ **C**   Ankle sprain
☐ **D**   Stress fracture of the tibia
☐ **E**   Tibialis posterior rupture

61 What is the best course of action for the management of this patient's leg pain?

☐ **A**   Refer to GP
☐ **B**   Supply paracetamol
☐ **C**   Supply paracetamol and NSAIDs
☐ **D**   Supply paracetamol and NSAIDs, and refer to GP
☐ **E**   None of the above

62 A 55-year-old patient with heart failure has just had an abdominal laparoscopic surgery which went well. Prior to surgery he took bisoprolol, spironolactone and furosemide. He has been nil-to-mouth and on IV fluids for the last couple of days. The following show his blood results on the third day on the ward:

	Value	Normal range
Sodium	135 mmol/L	137–144 mmol/L
Potassium	6.7 mmol/L	3.5–4.9 mmol/L
Chloride	95 mmol/L	95–107 mmol/L
Bicarbonate	28 mmol/L	20–28 mmol/L
Urea	9.8 mmol/L	2.5–7.5 mmol/L
Creatinine	101 mmol/L	60–110 mmol/L

What is the most likely cause of these results?

☐ **A**   Acute renal failure
☐ **B**   Adrenocortical failure
☐ **C**   Inadequate blood sample
☐ **D**   Liver toxicity
☐ **E**   Spironolactone therapy

63 A 40-year-old man presents to your diabetes clinic for an initial review. After some measurements you see that he has a normal BP and is obese. He also has glucose in his urine sample. You ask for his HbA1c levels and they come back at a level of 45 mmol/mol.

What is the most appropriate initial management option for this man?

- ☐ **A** Admit to hospital for insulin therapy
- ☐ **B** Advise on diet and exercise
- ☐ **C** Metformin treatment
- ☐ **D** Start insulin therapy
- ☐ **E** Sulphonylurea treatment

64 You are working on the adult post-surgical ward and have come to know that six patients and three members of staff on the ward have developed acute diarrhoea, nausea and vomiting over the past 24 hours. Which single virus is most likely to be responsible?

- ☐ **A** Adenovirus
- ☐ **B** Astrovirus
- ☐ **C** Enterovirus
- ☐ **D** Norovirus
- ☐ **E** Rotavirus

65 A 21-year-old asthmatic woman has worsening breathlessness and wheezing over 24 hours.
Which single investigation would be the most helpful in her initial management?

- ☐ **A** Chest X-ray
- ☐ **B** Full blood count
- ☐ **C** Peak expiratory flow rate
- ☐ **D** Serum concentration of potassium
- ☐ **E** Sputum culture

66 A new blood test has been developed to detect condition W. It was tested on 200 people; 100 people tested positive for W and 95 actually had the condition, while 5 people tested negative for the condition but were actually found to have the condition. The remainder who tested negative were found not to have the condition.
What is the negative predictive value of the test?

- ☐ **A** 5%
- ☐ **B** 10%
- ☐ **C** 50%
- ☐ **D** 95%
- ☐ **E** 100%

67 A 40-year-old man with a BMI of 32 is found to have a HbA1c level
of 52 mmol/mol. He has previously been advised to change his diet and
to exercise more often. However, there is a persistence of HbA1c level
above 50 mmol/mol. He has normal renal and liver function.
What is the most appropriate drug treatment for this patient?

    □ **A**   Acarbose
    □ **B**   Gliclazide
    □ **C**   Insulin glargine
    □ **D**   Metformin
    □ **E**   Rosiglitazone

68 An 18-month-old toddler with a nut allergy, who weighs 10 kg, has
presented to A & E with an anaphylactic reaction.
What dose of intramuscular adrenaline would you prescribe for this
child for use in an emergency?

    □ **A**   Adrenaline 100 micrograms
    □ **B**   Adrenaline 150 micrograms
    □ **C**   Adrenaline 250 micrograms
    □ **D**   Adrenaline 300 micrograms
    □ **E**   Adrenaline 500 micrograms

69 You are reading the notes of a cancer patient and notice that they have
been prescribed vinblastine.
Which route of administration should vinblastine ONLY ever be given?

    □ **A**   Intramuscularly
    □ **B**   Intrathecally
    □ **C**   Intravenously
    □ **D**   Oral
    □ **E**   Subcutaneously

70 Which of the following foods are NOT recommended for pregnant
women?

    □ **A**   Hard cheeses
    □ **B**   Nuts
    □ **C**   Red meats
    □ **D**   Soft blue cheeses
    □ **E**   Yoghurts

Extended matching questions

Sonia Kauser

> In this section, for each numbered question, select the one lettered option that most closely corresponds to the answer. Within each group of questions each lettered option may be used once, more than once or not at all.

Drug reactions

A	Hypercalcaemia
B	Hyperglycaemia
C	Hyperkalaemia
D	Hypernatraemia
E	Hypocalcaemia
F	Hypoglycaemia
G	Hypokalaemia
H	Hyponatraemia

> For questions 1–5
>
> For the patients described below, select the single most likely adverse drug reaction from the list above. Each option may be used once, more than once, or not at all

1   An elderly patient, aged 82, is admitted into an elderly medical admissions ward due to confusion, dizziness and tiredness. Her repeat prescription medication includes metformin, gliclazide, bisoprolol, clopidogrel and atorvastatin.

2   A patient, aged 42, has been admitted onto a medical admissions ward due to severe electrolyte imbalance which has continued despite correcting dehydration first. Drugs which inhibit the mobilisation of this electrolyte are usually used to manage the imbalance. A bisphosphonate such as pamidronate has been recommended to correct the patient's levels.

3   Mr AB, aged 77, has been admitted into a medical admissions ward with confusion, sickness, headaches and muscular ache. Upon admission you note the patient has recently been prescribed fluoxetine 20 mg OD, which was started 3 weeks ago.

4   Mr GC, aged 43, has recently started enalapril 10 mg OD for hypertension. He complains of an unusual heartbeat and muscular cramps that also feel like muscle weakness.

5   Mrs FT, aged 62, has a history of hepatic failure and the initiation of furosemide 20 mg OD has precipitated encephalopathy.

Skin

A   Acne vulgaris
B   Chicken pox
C   Eczema
D   Impetigo
E   Psoriasis
F   Shingles
G   Tinea corporis
H   Tinea pedis

For questions 6–10

For the patients described below, select the single most likely condition from the list above. Each option may be used once, more than once or not at all.

6   Mr GB, aged 22, presents to the community pharmacy with red, flaky, crusty patches of skin and they are covered in silvery scales.

7   Mr DT, aged 39, presents to the community pharmacy with itchy white patches between his toes and parts have become red, sore and flaky.

8   Miss BM, aged 34, presents to the community pharmacy with a tingling, painful, red and blotchy rash on the right side of her back. Some of the rash has formed blisters which are oozing fluid.

9   Miss TV, aged 21, presents to the community pharmacy with predominantly non-inflamed lesions (open and closed comedones) and few inflammatory lesions that are present on the face, back and chest.

10   Master AR, aged 5, presents to the community pharmacy with itchy, dry, cracked and sore skin. The inside of the elbows and the back of the knees are predominantly affected. He has a past medical history of asthma.

Eye

A   Allergic conjunctivitis
B   Bacterial conjunctivitis
C   Dry eye
D   Glaucoma
E   Keratitis
F   Subconjunctival haemorrhage
G   Uveitis
H   Viral conjunctivitis

For questions 11–15

For the patients described below, select the single most likely condition from the list above. Each option may be used once, more than once or not at all.

11   Mr GK, aged 61, wishes to discuss a recent diagnosis with you in the pharmacy. He informs you that the specialist informed him this condition developed slowly and was picked up during a routine eye test (raised pressure). He has experienced some blurred vision and noticed rainbow coloured circles around very bright lights.

12   Mr BA, aged 38, presents to the community pharmacy and is very concerned regarding his red eye. He woke up this morning and noticed redness on his sclera. He is currently in no pain and not aware of any discharge from either eye.

13 Mrs FM, aged 42, presents to the community pharmacy complaining of a dull ache around her left eye which is worse on focusing. She reports photophobia, blurry vision and also noticed 'small shapes' moving across her vision. The symptoms developed suddenly.

14 Mr HN, aged 21, presents to the community pharmacy with sore itchy eyes. He informs you of watery discharge affecting both eyes. He has no other symptoms. His past medical history includes asthma and eczema.

15 Miss AN, aged 28, presents to the community pharmacy with sore, gritty eyes. Upon waking she has noticed yellow/green pus causing her eyelashes to stick together. Both eyes are affected. No pain is reported.

Diabetes medication

    A   Empagliflozin
    B   Gliclazide
    C   Glucagon
    D   Isophane insulin
    E   Linagliptin
    F   Metformin
    G   Pioglitazone
    H   Replaglinide

For questions 16–20

For the patients described below, select the single most likely medication from the list above. Each option may be used once, more than once or not at all.

16 Mrs MK, aged 32, is 28 weeks pregnant and diagnosed with gestational diabetes. She has a raised fasting glucose (7 mmol/L), and her midwife and consultant have agreed to start her on immediate therapy. Metformin is not suitable for Mrs MK.

17 Mr CP, aged 45, has been diagnosed with type 2 diabetes and is being commenced on monotherapy due to raised HbA1c (52 mmol/mol). He has a BMI of 30 kg/m^2.

18 Mrs JR, aged 48, has been diagnosed with type 2 diabetes and is being commenced on monotherapy due to raised HbA1c (52 mmol/mol). She has a BMI of 18 kg/m^2.

19 Mr AP, aged 62, requires an additional oral agent due to his poorly controlled type 2 diabetes. His diabetic nurse avoids this medication as Mr AP has a history of bladder cancer.

20 Mr RT, aged 59, has been started on a new medication for her type 2 diabetes. You decide to counsel this patient on a dangerous side effect. You advise Mr RT to seek urgent medical advice if he ever experiences severe pain, tenderness or swelling in his genital area, particularly if it is accompanied by a fever or tiredness.

Cardiovascular medication

- A   Apixaban PO
- B   Aspirin PO
- C   Clopidogrel PO
- D   Dalteparin SC
- E   Phytomenadione IV
- F   Rivaroxaban PO
- G   Ticagrelor PO
- H   Warfarin PO

For questions 21–25

For the patients described below, select the single most likely medication from the list above. Each option may be used once, more than once or not at all.

21 Mr KL, aged 62, following his NSTEMI will now be prescribed this medication long term. He has no known allergies or intolerances.

22 Mrs FB, aged 58, following a stroke will now be prescribed this medication long term. She has no known allergies or intolerances.

23 Mr GB, aged 65, has valvular atrial fibrillation and requires long-term anticoagulation.

24 Miss SP, aged 30, has been diagnosed with a deep vein thrombosis and is currently 21 weeks pregnant. She requires treatment.

25 Mr VP, aged 52, has non valvular atrial fibrillation and requires anticoagulation. He has a past medical history of antiphospholipid syndrome.

Antibiotics

  A   Amoxicillin
  B   Cefalexin
  C   Doxycycline
  D   Flucloxacillin
  E   Gentamicin
  F   Lymecycline
  G   Metronidazole
  H   Trimethoprim

For questions 26–30

For the patients described below, select the single most likely medication from the list above. Each option may be used once, more than once or not at all.

26 Mr TK, aged 38, has been diagnosed with Lyme disease and it is recommended to prescribe the suggested first-line treatment. He has no known allergies or intolerances.

27 Miss SB, aged 23, has been diagnosed with an uncomplicated UTI and it is recommended to prescribe the suggested first-line treatment. She has no known past medical history, allergies or intolerances. She is not pregnant.

28 Miss SL, aged 26, has been diagnosed with bacterial vaginosis and it is recommended to prescribe the suggested first-line treatment. She has no known past medical history, allergies or intolerances. She is not pregnant.

29 Mr FB, aged 31, has been diagnosed with acute cellulitis on his left leg and it is recommended to prescribe the suggested first-line treatment. He has no known past medical history, allergies or intolerances.

30 Mr KW, aged 46, has been diagnosed with community-acquired pneumonia. His CURB score is 0 and it has been decided to manage him at home due to low severity. He has no known past medical history, allergies or intolerances.

Antibiotic side effects

  A   Cefalexin
  B   Ciprofloxacin
  C   Clarithromycin

D   Co-amoxiclav
E   Flucloxacillin
F   Gentamicin
G   Nitrofurantoin
H   Tetracycline

For questions 31–35

For the patients described below, select the single most likely adverse drug reaction from the list above. Each option may be used once, more than once or not at all.

31 Mr GT, aged 52, has been prescribed this antibiotic for over two weeks. Cholestatic jaundice and hepatitis can rarely occur with this antibiotic. This needs to be prescribed cautiously due to his history of hepatic impairment.

32 Miss HJ, aged 11, has been offered this medication to manage her acne, however you note that this is not suitable for her due to a risk of staining and dental hypoplasia.

33 Mr CP, aged 69, has been prescribed this for pneumonia whilst in hospital. Ototoxicity and nephrotoxicity have been reported with this medication.

34 Mrs PL, aged 58, has been prescribed this medication for hospital-acquired pneumonia. Care needs to be taken when co-prescribed with her usual simvastatin.

35 Mr DL, aged 61, has been prescribed this medication, however since initiation he reports heel pain. Upon reviewing, you decide this may not be safe to continue.

Antidepressant medication

A   Amitriptyline
B   Fluoxetine
C   Lithium
D   Lofepramine
E   Mirtazapine
F   Paroxetine
G   Sertraline
H   Venlafaxine

For questions 36–40

For the patients described below, select the single most likely medication from the list above. Each option may be used once, more than once or not at all.

36 Mrs MS, aged 58, has been prescribed this antidepressant for her major depression. She will require regular BP monitoring as she has a history of hypertension and heart disease.

37 Mr MR, aged 35, has noticed an increased appetite and also weight gain since the initiation of his new medication.

38 Miss BN, aged 52, has overdosed on this medication and is admitted onto the medical admissions award. The senior pharmacist informs you that this medication belongs to tricyclic and related antidepressants and is associated with the lowest risk of fatality in overdose.

39 Mr MI, aged 67, has recently had a myocardial infarction and also has a history of angina symptoms. This antidepressant is chosen as it is known to be safe.

40 Mrs SR, aged 48, has been prescribed this medication for her recurrent depression. Regular drug level monitoring is recommended.

Antihypertensive medication
- A Amlodipine
- B Bisoprolol
- C Candesartan
- D Chlortalidone
- E Indapamide
- F Labetalol
- G Lisinopril
- H Verapamil

For questions 41–45

For the patients described below, select the single most likely medication from the list above. Each option may be used once, more than once or not at all.

41 Mr GP, aged 58, has been prescribed this medication, however you note he is also prescribed carvedilol and advise against prescribing this medication due to a risk of cardiovascular side effects.

42 Mrs NP, aged 56, has been diagnosed with stage 1 hypertension. She is of south Asian background. She has no known allergies and drug intolerances. She is prescribed the recommended first-line treatment.

43 Mrs RN, aged 28, has been diagnosed with gestational hypertension. She is to commence on the first-line recommended therapy.

44 Mrs LA, aged 58, has type 2 diabetes and has recently been diagnosed with hypertension. This medication has been selected in order to delay progression of microalbuminuria to nephropathy.

45 Mrs CP, aged 63, has type 2 diabetes and also hypertension. This medication is generally avoided as it can mask the symptoms of hypoglycaemia.

Scoring classifications

A $CHA_2 DS_2$-VASc score
B Cholesterol test
C Creatinine clearance
D FeverPAIN score
E HAS-BLED score
F QRISK calculator
G TTR (Time in therapeutic range)
H UKMEC score

For questions 46–50

For the examples described below, select the single most likely test from the list above. Each option may be used once, more than once or not at all.

46 A patient presents to your minor ailments' clinic within the GP surgery. They present complaining of sore throat symptoms. This classification helps determine how to manage this patient.

47 A classification to determine if a patient requires anticoagulation.

48 A score to measure the anticoagulation control of warfarin therapy.

49 An investigation to determine the maintenance dose of rivaroxaban being prescribed for the prevention of stroke.

50 A classification in order to aid the prescribing decisions for contraceptive methods.

SECTION B

Oksana Pyzik

In this section, for each numbered question, select the one lettered option that most closely corresponds to the answer. Within each group of questions each lettered option may be used once, more than once or not at all.

Parasitic infections

A *Blastocystis hominis*
B *Dientamoeba fragilis*
C *Enterobius vermicularis*
D *Giardia lamblia*
E *Pediculus humanus capitis*
F *Sarcoptes scabiei*
G *Toxoplasma gondii*
H *Trichomonas vaginalis*

For questions 1–8

For the scenarios described below, select the single most likely responsible parasite from the list above. Each option may be used once, more than once, or not at all.

1   A 44-year-old male presents at the clinic with complaints of pro-fuse, watery diarrhoea, anorexia, abdominal pain and cramping, and increased eructation over the past 5 weeks. He has a significantly decreased appetite and eating appears to exacerbate his symptoms. He described his stools as greasy, foul-smelling but he had not seen any blood, mucus, or pus in his stools. He reported a weight loss of approx-imately 5 kg over the past 3 weeks. He has not recently travelled outside of the UK. The GP ordered a laboratory test which came back positive for the most common cause of infectious gastroenteritis worldwide. The patient was prescribed *Flagyl*® 250 mg by mouth three times per day for 7 days.

2   A 7-year-old female complains of an itchy scalp and the mother reports that the girl appears to have developed dandruff.

3   The parasite lays anywhere from 50–150 eggs during her 30–40-day lifespan.

4   A 20-year-old female has recently had unprotected intercourse and presents with lower abdominal pain and dysuria.

5   A 23-year-old male complains of intense pruritus around the genitals which worsens at night.

6   A patient is prescribed permethrin 5% cream (washed off after 8 to 12 hours) and crotamiton 10% cream to treat this condition.

7   A 5-year-old child presents with perianal pruritus at night.

8   A 53-year-old male presents with flu-like symptoms, swollen lymph glands, muscle aches and pains that have lasted for 2 months. He owns three cats and lives alone.

Vaccines

A   Human papillomavirus vaccine
B   Influenza vaccine
C   MMR vaccine
D   Pertussis vaccine
E   Pneumococcal vaccine
F   Rotavirus vaccine
G   Varicella vaccine
H   Yellow fever vaccine

For questions 9–13

For the scenarios described below, select the single most likely vaccine that fits the description from the list above. Each option may be used once, more than once or not at all.

9   Is not offered to children via the NHS due to concerns that it could increase the risk of shingles in adults.

10 Protects against genital warts.

11 Recommended for patients who have had their spleen removed.

12 Offered to pregnant women to protect them and their babies against whooping cough.

13 The first oral dose is given to infants at 8 weeks.

Oncology

    A   5-fluorouracil
    B   Anastrozole
    C   Bleomycin
    D   Cisplatin
    E   Dexamethasone
    F   Ondansetron
    G   Tamoxifen
    H   Trastuzumab

> **For questions 14–22**
>
> For the scenarios described below, select the single most likely treatment from the list above. Each option may be used once, more than once or not at all.

14 A 70-year-old male has commenced treatment for stage 3 colon cancer and suffers from severe nausea and vomiting. He has been prescribed a $5HT_3$ receptor antagonist to inhibit the chemoreceptor trigger zone (CZT) vomiting centre.

15 Is prescribed as an adjunct to manage symptoms of nausea and vomiting.

16 May cause palmar-plantar erythrodysesthaesia.

17 A 50-year-old female has HER2 positive metastatic breast cancer.

18 May be prescribed for the primary prevention of breast cancer in women at moderate or high risk.

19 A two- to three-fold increase in the risk for VTE has been demonstrated in healthy women.

20 Careful monitoring by audiometry should be performed prior to initiation of therapy and prior to subsequent doses.

21 Treatment should be stopped at the first sign of oral ulceration, or if there is evidence of gastrointestinal side effects such as stomatitis, diarrhoea, bleeding from the gastrointestinal tract of haemorrhage at any site, oesophagopharyngitis or intractable vomiting.

22 Should not be used in premenopausal women with breast cancer.

Dermatology

A Amorolfine
B Benzoyl peroxide
C Co-cypyrindiol
D Hydrocortisone
E Isotretinoin
F Ketoconazole
G Metronidazole
H Selenium sulphide

For questions 23–31

For the scenarios described below, select the single most likely treatment from the list above. Each option may be used once, more than once or not at all.

23 A 41-year-old female presents with pustules and papules, erythema, flushed cheeks, dry eyes and rhinophyma.

24 A 19-year-old male wants to purchase this medicine over the counter but first wants to know how it works. As the pharmacist you explain that this topically applied medical product reduces the local population of *Propionibacterium,* leading to a reduction in the production of irritant fatty acids in the sebaceous glands.

25 A 21-year-old female with moderate acne has discontinued this medicine 3 months after her acne has been controlled.

26 A 25-year-old male presents with onychomycosis on the toenails of his right foot. As the pharmacist you recommend an over-the-counter product and instruct to apply to the affected toenails once weekly.

27 A 54-year-old female presents with dandruff. As the pharmacist, you recommend a product that acts as an antiseborrhoeic agent which effectively controls itching and scaling dandruff through its cytostatic effect on cells of the epidermis and follicular epithelium, thus reducing corneocyte production.

28 A 23-year-old male presents with pityriasis versicolor. As the pharmacist, you recommend a product that is a synthetic imidazole-dioxalane derivative. It has broad spectrum antifungal activity which inhibits the growth of common dermatophytes and yeasts by altering the permeability of the cell membrane.

29 A 25-year-old female presents at the pharmacy to collect her prescription 14 days after it was issued. As the pharmacist you explain that you are unable to dispense this medication because it must be dispensed within 7 days of the prescription issue date. You explain to the patient that a new prescription is required.

30 A 19-year-old male is prescribed a new treatment. He must have his serum lipids (fasting values) checked before treatment, 1 month after the start of treatment, and subsequently at 3-monthly intervals.

31 A 44-year-old male is prescribed a topical cream for moderate eczema and asks about side effects. As the pharmacist you explain that it is generally well tolerated but should be applied thinly as may cause thinning of the skin and striae, but to stop treatment immediately if an allergic reaction occurs.

Cardiovascular health

A   Amiodarone
B   Aspirin
C   Cangrelor
D   Clopidogrel
E   Digoxin
F   Furosemide
G   Ramipril
H   Simvastatin

For questions 32–37

For the scenarios described below, select the single most likely treatment from the list above. Each option may be used once, more than once or not at all.

32 The maintenance dosage should be based upon the percentage of the peak body stores lost each day through elimination.

33 May cause creatine kinase to rise above ten times the upper limit of normal. Thus, certain groups such as women and the elderly (age $\geq$ 65 years) should have their CK level measured before starting treatment.

34 A 77-year-old male presents with acute heart failure and dyspnoea due to pulmonary congestion.

35 Is co-administered with acetylsalicylic acid (ASA) and is indicated for the reduction of thrombotic cardiovascular events in adult patients with coronary artery disease undergoing percutaneous coronary intervention (PCI) who have not received an oral P2Y12 inhibitor prior to the PCI procedure.

36 Is a cardiac glycoside that increases the force of myocardial contraction and reduces conductivity within the atrioventricular (AV) node.

37 A 56-year-old male with atrial fibrillation has been taking his medication for several years. However, recently he complains of weight gain and cold intolerance. Upon clinical examination excessive bradycardia is discovered and further tests reveal an increase in serum usTSH and an exaggerated TSH response to TRH and low T3 and T4 levels.

Pathogens

A *Bordetella pertussis*
B *Epstein-Barr virus*
C *Escherichia coli*
D *Klebsiella pneumoniae*
E *Methicillin-resistant Staphylococcus aureus*
F *Moraxella catarrhalis*
G *Mycobacterium tuberculosis*
H *Respiratory syncytial virus*

For questions 38–44

For the scenarios described below, select the single most likely responsible pathogen from the list above. Each option may be used once, more than once or not at all.

38 A patient presents with cough that has lasted 6 weeks and suffers from night sweats. You are required to report this to the local authority proper officers under the Health Protection (Notification) Regulations 2010.

39 Is more commonly found in elderly people who have had contact with healthcare services - they can present in hospital or in the community.

40 Is a gram-negative, aerobic, oxidase-positive diplococcus that commonly causes otitis media in children.

41 A 3-month-old infant contracts a cough that is characterised by paroxysms which are consist of a short expiratory burst followed by an inspiratory gasp.

42 Is a single-stranded, negative-sense ribonucleic acid (RNA) virus and a member of the *Pneumoviridae* family that causes lower respiratory tract infections in children and complications can lead to bronchiolitis.

43 Easily spreads through the saliva, often presenting as typical flu-like symptoms along with possible swollen glands and a rash.

44 A 19-year-old female presents with symptoms of dysuria, haematuria and increased urinary frequency.

Paediatrics

    A   Chicken pox
    B   Glandular fever
    C   Impetigo
    D   Measles
    E   Meningitis
    F   Molluscum contagiosum
    G   Mumps
    H   Reye's syndrome

For questions 45–50

For the scenarios described below, select the single most likely condition from the list above. Each option may be used once, more than once or not at all.

45 Five days ago, a 12-year-old female experienced flu-like symptoms including high fever. Since then she has been admitted to hospital after suffering a seizure and is continuously vomiting. A blood test shows that her blood sugar level has dropped, while ammonia levels have increased up to 1.5 times the normal level. The patient requires a lumbar puncture to confirm diagnosis. Upon reviewing the patient's medication history with her mother, you suggest to the consultant that the condition may be drug induced.

46 A 6-month-old infant is refusing to feed, has a slight bulge protruding from the top of their head and is making jerky movements along with grunting sounds. The mother is very concerned as these symptoms appeared suddenly.

47 A mother collects a prescription for topical fusidic acid for her 2-year-old child. As the pharmacist you instruct that the cream should be applied three times a day for 5 days.

48 A 14-year-old boy presents with small dome-shaped, pearly white papules with a central umbilication that are clustered across his trunk and flexures.

49 A 16-year-old male complains of constant fatigue, headache, persistent sore throat, and tender, swollen lymph glands.

50 A 4-year-old child presents with a fever and small, bluish-white spots with a red ring along the palate as shown in the image below.

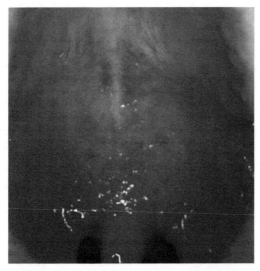

Source: https://www.cdc.gov/measles/symptoms/photos.html

SECTION C

Pratik Thakkar

In this section, for each numbered question, select the one lettered option that most closely corresponds to the answer. Within each group of questions each lettered option may be used once, more than once or not at all.

Evidence based medicine

A   <0.00001
B   0.0002
C   1
D   5.13
E   5.42
F   102
G   169
H   569
I   1057
J   1537

For questions 1–5

For the statements described below, select the single most likely option from the list above. Each option may be used once, more than once, or not at all.

The diagram shows a forest plot for three randomised trials which compared the risk of hypoglycaemia for type 2 diabetes patients treated with metformin + sulphonylurea (M+S) versus those treated with metformin + GLP-1 inhibitors (M+G).

Study or subgroup	Metformin plus sulphonylurea n/N	Metformin plus GLP-I n/N	Risk Ratio M-H, Random, 95% CI	Weight	Risk Ratio M-H, Random, 95% CI
Ahr n 2014	102/307	35/302		32.4 %	2.87 [2.02, 4.07]
Gallwitz 2012a (I)	240/508	102/511		37.2 %	2.37 [1.94, 2.88]
Nauck 2013 (2)	58/242	32/724		30.4 %	5.42 [3.61, 8.14]
Total (95% CI)	**1057**	**1537**		**100.0%**	**3.24 [2.05, 5.13]**

Total events: 400 (Metformin plus sulphonylurea), 169 (Metformin plus GLP-I)
Heterogeneity: Tau^2 = 0.14; Chi^2 = 12.99, df = 2 (P = 0.002); I^2 = 85%
Test for overall effect: Z = 5.02 (P < 0.00001)
Test for subgroup differences: Not applicable

0.05 0.2   1   5   20
Favours metformin + sulphonylurea   Favours metformin + GLP-I

Source: https://www.cochranelibrary.com/cdsr/doi/10.1002/14651858.CD012368.pub2/full)

1   The expected value of the risk ratio if hypoglycaemic episodes were equally likely to occur for patients treated with M+S group versus those in the M+G group.

2   The upper confidence limit when information from all studies were combined.

3   The best estimate of the risk ratio from the Nauck 2013 study.

4   The p value when comparing incidence of hypoglycaemic episodes between M+S group and M+G group in this review.

5   The total number of events across both groups in this review.

Anticoagulation

A   Activated partial thromboplastin time (APTT)
B   Aspirin
C   Dipyridamole
D   Enoxaparin
E   Full blood count
F   Imipramine
G   International normalised ratio (INR)
H   Liver function test
I   Vitamin K
J   Warfarin

For questions 6–10

For the patient described below, select the single most likely option from the list above. Each option may be used once, more than once, or not at all.

A 55-year-old woman presents with suspected deep vein thrombosis. She presents to the A & E department.

6   The most appropriate drug to give her immediately before any further tests are confirmed.

7   The best product to give for longer term management.

8   The OTC drug that is likely to increase the risk of bleeding with warfarin.

9   The patient misread the label of a warfarin treatment course and is now over anticoagulated. This medicine should be offered as an antidote.

10 If on warfarin, the usual way to monitor the patient's anticoagulation.

Hay fever
   A   Beclometasone
   B   Cetirizine
   C   Diphenhydramine
   D   Hydrocortisone
   E   Inhalation
   F   Intranasal
   G   Oral
   H   Phenylephrine
   I   Sodium cromoglicate
   J   Theophylline

For questions 11–15

For the patient described below, select the single most likely treatment from the list above. Each option may be used once, more than once, or not at all.

An 18-year-old high school student suffers from hay fever and has presented to your pharmacy with an exacerbation of her hay fever symptoms.

11 The patient would like to have a medication that doesn't interfere with her daily activities. Select an appropriate antihistamine with which to start treatment.

12 The route of administration that is most appropriate for over-the-counter treatment of hay fever.

13 The student finds that the antihistamine cetirizine does not control the symptoms well. Select an anti-inflammatory drug for further treatment.

14 The best route of administering a steroid for treatment of hay fever.

15 The patient has complained of nasal congestion. This medication can be offered to relieve congestion of the nasal passage.

Healthcare statistics

    A   Bias
    B   Blinding
    C   Concealment of allocation
    D   Confidence interval (CI)
    E   Heterogeneity
    F   Homogeneity
    G   Kappa
    H   Number needed to harm (NNH)
    I   Number needed to treat (NNT)
    J   Pooled analysis

For questions 16–20

For the definitions described below, select the single most likely term from the list above. Each option may be used once, more than once, or not at all.

16 The number of patients who require a new intervention to prevent a single adverse outcome.

17 The range within which the true value of a population parameter might lie.

18 A combined summary of results from several studies of a particular topic.

19 Systematic (as opposed to random) deviation of the results of a study from the 'true' results, which is caused by the way the study is designed or conducted.

20 A way to prevent researchers, doctors and patients in a clinical trial from knowing which study group each patient is in so they cannot influence the results.

Dosing regimens

    A   Daily
    B   Twice a day
    C   5 days
    D   Once a week
    E   Biweekly
    F   28 days
    G   1 month
    H   6 months
    I   180 days
    J   None of the above

For questions 21–25

For the statements described below, select the single most likely time interval from the list above. Each option may be used once, more than once or not at all.

21 The amount of time a regular (non-controlled drug) NHS prescription is valid for from the date of signature from the prescriber.

22 The maximum validity of a schedule 2 and schedule 3 controlled drug prescription.

23 Methotrexate is usually given at this time interval for management of rheumatoid arthritis.

24 Folic acid 400 mcg is recommended at this dosing interval for women wanting to get pregnant.

25 In an emergency supply setting, the maximum supply of phenobarbital for patients.

Hormones

  A   Androgen
  B   Catecholamine
  C   Eicosanoids
  D   Fat soluble vitamin
  E   Glucocorticoid
  F   Mineralocorticoid
  G   Oestrogen
  H   Peptide hormone
  I   Progestogen
  J   Thyroid hormone

For questions 26–30

For the hormones described below, select the single most likely class of hormone from the list above. Each option may be used once, more than once or not at all.

26 Aldosterone.

27 Estradiol.

28 Progesterone.

29 Thyroxine.

30 Cortisol.

Calculation questions

Ryan Hamilton

1   Mr A comes into your pharmacy with a prescription for his 4-year-old son who has been prescribed flucloxacillin 125 mg/5 mL suspension at a dose of 125 mg QDS for 5 days.

Given that when 100 mL of the suspension is made up it has an expiry date of 7 days, how many bottles should you supply? Give your answer to the nearest whole number.

2   Mrs B is due to commence a course of chemotherapy for leukaemia, and the consultants would like to treat her with daunorubicin dosed by body surface area at 45 mg/m^2. You look at Mrs H's notes and find that she is 1.48 m tall and weighs 72 kg.

Calculate the dose of daunorubicin to the nearest 5 mg. Give your answer to the nearest whole number.

Mosteller formula for calculating body surface area:

$$BSA(m^2) = ([\text{height (cm)} \times \text{weight (kg)}] \div 3600)^{0.5}$$

3   Mrs C has been diagnosed with an acute flare of ulcerative colitis and has been prescribed prednisolone. You are given her prescription and note she has been placed on a weaning dose of prednisolone. She is required to take a high dose of prednisolone 60 mg OD for 6 more days then wean by 5 mg every week, then stop.

How many 5 mg prednisolone tablets should you supply to ensure Mrs C can complete her course? Give your answer to the nearest whole number.

4   Mr D has been newly diagnosed with pulmonary MDR-TB and his medical team are going to add in prothionamide 15 mg/kg once daily to his treatment regimen. On the ward round you note that Mr D weighs 56 kg and has an eGFR of greater than 90 mL/min. You

consult the TB drug monographs website (www.tbdrugmonographs
.co.uk) and find the following information for prothionamide:

PROTHIONAMIDE

Please note prothionamide is not licensed in the UK.

Prothionamide is a thioamide and is considered to be interchangeable
with ethionamide (currently not available in the UK).

DOSAGE

Adult & paediatric doses are the same per kg.

Adults: 15-20 mg/kg (max. 1 g) once daily (oral).

Once daily dosing is preferred to maximise peak levels, particularly for
daily doses ≤750 mg. Consider twice daily dosing if patients are unable
to tolerate once daily regimens.

Children: 15-20 mg/kg (max. 1 g) once daily (oral).

Once daily dosing is preferred to maximise peak levels, particularly for
daily doses ≤750 mg. Consider twice daily dosing if patients are unable
to tolerate once daily regimens.

WHO advise a once daily dosing regimen if tolerated (to maximise
peak levels), but twice daily regimens may be required if unable to
tolerate.

Prothionamide should be taken with or after meals to reduce gastrointestinal adverse effects. Most patients also require gradual dose
escalation, i.e. for adults: initially 250 mg once a day, increasing by
250 mg every 3 to 5 days.

All patients must be prescribed pyridoxine whilst receiving prothionamide. The usual adult dose ranges from 50 to 100 mg daily, up to 50 mg
per 250 mg of prothionamide.

PREPARATIONS

Oral: 250 mg tablets (unlicensed medicine).

Knowing that the tablets can be split in half, what total daily dose
should the medical team prescribe for Mr D? Give your answer to
the nearest whole number.

5   Mrs E has been admitted to your ward and has had a nasogastric tube fitted. While undertaking her medication history you note she was taking phenytoin capsules 300 mg twice daily to control her epilepsy. You advise the medical team to prescribe the oral suspension of phenytoin to be given down the nasogastric tube.

How many millilitres of phenytoin oral suspension should Mrs E be given for each dose? Give your answer to the nearest whole millilitre. You may use the phenytoin monograph in the BNF to help you.

6   Mr F is a gentleman who has been taking carbamazepine 400 mg BD, as modified-release tablets, for his epilepsy. He has been admitted to your hospital after suffering an ischaemic stroke and you advise to change his carbamazepine to suppositories until his swallowing improves.

What dose of carbamazepine suppositories would you advise to prescribe Mr F for each individual dose? Give your answer to the nearest whole milligram.

You may use the carbamazepine monograph in the BNF to help you.

7   You receive a prescription for Miss G who is being newly started on gabapentin for neuropathic pain. The prescription is for the standard induction regimen of 300 mg OD on day 1, then 300 mg BD on day 2, and then 300 mg TDS thereafter.

How many gabapentin 300 mg capsules do you need to dispense if the total duration on the prescription is 28 days? Give your answer to the nearest whole number.

8   Mr H is one of your cystic fibrosis patients and is being discharged on IV ceftazidime 2 g every 12 hours, to be administered through the local outpatient parenteral antibiotic therapy (OPAT) scheme. Each ceftazidime 2 g vial is reconstituted with 10 mL sodium chloride 0.9% and given as a bolus. The nurses will also flush the patient's line with 10 mL sodium chloride 0.9% before and after each dose is given.

How many 10 mL sodium chloride 0.9% ampoules should be supplied to sufficiently cover a 6-week course? Round up your answer to the nearest 5 ampoules to enable easy supply.

9   Mrs I is required to take co-trimoxazole for prophylaxis against *Pneumocystis jirovecii* (*Pneumocystis carinii*) infections at a dose of 960 mg each morning and evening on Mondays, Wednesdays and Fridays. Your pharmacy only stocks the 480 mg strength of co-trimoxazole.

How many 480 mg co-trimoxazole tablets are you required to cover a 26-week (6-month) period? Give your answer to the nearest whole number.

10   Mr J is taking warfarin for a prosthetic heart valve and has just been to the anticoagulation clinic to get his INR checked. He presents you with his yellow book which advises Mr J to take 3 mg every day except Sunday and Wednesday when he will take 4 mg. Your hospital's outpatient clinic policy is to use 1 mg tablets only.

How many packs of twenty-eight warfarin 1 mg tablets do you need to supply for 4 weeks? Give your answer to the nearest whole pack to provide sufficient doses.

11   Mrs C is a patient on your nutrition ward who has a long-term Hickman line in place for the administration of parenteral nutrition. The Hickman line has become infected with coagulase-negative *Staphylococcus* and the medical team would like to treat this by using vancomycin line locks. The patient will be using 3 mL of a 100 mg/10 mL solution of vancomycin to dwell in the line for 24 hours before being changed. You advise the medical team that if the line lock is flushed into the patient this will need to be done slowly to avoid adverse reactions.

What is the shortest amount of time over which the vancomycin line locks can be flushed? Give your answer to the nearest whole minute. You may use the SPC for vancomycin to help you: https://www.medicines.org.uk/emc/product/649/smpc

12   Mr P has been admitted to your intensive care unit with sepsis. He is 62 years old, 6 feet tall and weighs 63.4 kg. Recent blood tests show his eGFR is currently reduced at 73 mL/minute, but his other electrolytes are normal. Two days later, the microbiology department has identified *Stenotrophomonas maltophilia* from the patient's blood cultures and would like to give IV co-trimoxazole to treat this. As Mr P is severely unwell, the microbiologist advises a dose of 15 mg/kg/day of the trimethoprim component given in three divided doses.

Calculate the dose of co-trimoxazole to be prescribed for Mr P for each individual dose. Give your answer to the nearest 96 mg, which is equivalent to 1 mL of the available IV co-trimoxazole product.

You may use the SPC for IV co-trimoxazole to help you: https://www.medicines.org.uk/emc/product/4669/smpc

13   Mr J is 21 years old, weighing 72 kg, and has just been admitted to your A & E with suspected paracetamol poisoning and the medical team would like you to find out how much paracetamol he has taken so they can initiate the correct treatment. When taking his medication history, you find he has taken two whole packs of co-codamol, which he bought over the counter, along with a whole bottle of vodka. His partner has brought in the packaging, which you see were packs of 30 tablets.
Calculate how many milligrams of paracetamol per kilogram of body weight has Mr J has taken in this overdose episode. Give your answer to the nearest whole milligram.

14   Mrs W, who weighs 98 kg and is 5′ 3″ tall, has been admitted to your ward with worsening pyelonephritis, which has caused sepsis. The medical team would like to add a STAT dose of gentamicin to her current antimicrobial regimen. You decide to dose the gentamicin at 7 mg/kg based on ideal body weight.
What dose of gentamicin should be prescribed for Mrs W? Give your answer to the nearest 40 mg.

Formula for estimating ideal body weight:

Male IBW = 50 kg + 2.3 kg for every inch over 5 feet in height

Female IBW = 45.5 kg + 2.3 kg for every inch over 5 feet in height

15   Mr G has been newly started on amiodarone by his cardiologist. He presents to your pharmacy with a prescription for amiodarone tablets 200 mg TDS for 1 week, then 200 mg BD for 1 week, then 200 mg OD thereafter. The cardiologist will be seeing Mr G in 4 weeks' time for a review.
How many amiodarone 200 mg tablets should be supplied to last until Mr G's next cardiology appointment? Give your answer to the nearest whole number.

16   You are a quality control pharmacist working in the QA and QC labs and you are testing the concentration of drug S in a batch of solution. Utilising UV-visible spectrophotometry at 255 nm you find the absorbance (A) to be 0.701. Your QC department has produced the following calibration curve for drug S.

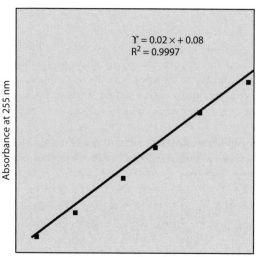

$$Y = 0.02 \times + 0.08$$
$$R^2 = 0.9997$$

Absorbance at 255 nm

Concentration of drug S (mg/mL)

Based on this absorbance result, calculate the concentration of drug S in the solution. Give your answer to two decimal places.

17   You are undertaking a quality improvement project to reduce waiting times in the pharmacy. In order to have a baseline to measure against you decide to calculate the current average waiting time. You obtain the following data from your system.

Patient	Waiting time (minutes)
AD	35
JG	45
LO	22
PD	34
BG	28
OO	54
LS	12
XS	33
WQ	36
FE	41

Calculate the mean average waiting time. Give your answer to the nearest whole minute.

18   Mr R has suffered from a severe cutaneous drug reaction and has been using *Emollin*® emollient spray. He is currently using two to three cans of *Emollin*® per day and needs another 3 weeks' treatment to last until his next dermatology appointment.

    How many cans of *Emollin*® emollient spray should be supplied to last until his next appointment? Give your answer to the nearest whole number.

19   Mr U, who weighs 76 kg, is being treated with IV teicoplanin to treat his osteomyelitis. He was initiated at a dose of 912 mg (equivalent to 12 mg/kg) once daily but his drug level has come back low at 16.3 mg/L. The consultant would like to achieve a level of at least 20 mg/L to ensure successful treatment.

    Calculate the minimum dose that should be prescribed for Mr U. Give your answer to the nearest 10 mg.

    You may use the SPC for IV teicoplanin to help you: https://www.medicines.org.uk/emc/product/2927/smpc

20   You have received a prescription for Mrs V, a 92-year-old lady who is receiving end of life care, is developing swallowing problems and has poor vascular access. Her consultant has written a prescription for twenty-eight (28) 1 g suppositories containing morphine sulfate 5 mg, which you will need to make up extemporaneously. You find the displacement value of morphine sulfate in Witepsol is 1.6 and you will need to make an excess of 1 suppository to ensure the order is filled. Calculate what mass of Witepsol you would need. Give your answer to three decimal places.

21   Mr S, who is 58 years old and weighs 64.6 kg, has been admitted to your ward, and the medical team would like to prescribe some routine intravenous maintenance fluids for him as he is unable to eat or drink.

    Calculate the minimum total volume of fluid that should be prescribed for Mr S over the course of the day. Give your answer to the nearest whole number.

    You may use the NICE Guideline for 'Intravenous fluid therapy in adults in hospital' to help you: https://www.nice.org.uk/guidance/cg174

22   Miss R is being treated for toxic epidermal necrolysis, possibly caused by ibuprofen. To provide nutritional support, the dietician would like to supplement Miss R with 1.5 g/kg/day of protein using *TwoCal*® liquid via a nasogastric tube. You find that Miss R weighs 52.8 kg.

What volume of *TwoCal*® liquid should be prescribed to meet Miss R's daily requirements? Give your answer to the nearest 10 millilitres. You may use Appendix 2: Borderline substances from the BNF to help you.

23   Bradley is a 3-month-old boy on your paediatric gastroenterology unit who is receiving parenteral nutrition. He has been reviewed by the nutrition team, who have altered his feeding regimen because he has gained weight. The volume of the aqueous proportion of the new parenteral nutrition regimen is 295 mL, which is to be run over 18 hours, each day.
What rate should the infusion pump be set to to deliver the parenteral nutrition over the required time period? Give your answer to one decimal place.

24   Mrs L is a 45-year-old lady who has just been admitted to your respiratory ward with a severe exacerbation of asthma. The admission clerking states she was weighed at 97 kg, her height is 5′ 4″, she smokes 10 cigarettes per day, drinks a little alcohol, but otherwise has no other comorbidities or allergies. The medical team want to start Mrs L on an infusion of aminophylline.
What dose of aminophylline infusion should be prescribed as the loading dose for Mrs L? Give your answer to the nearest whole number.
You may use this excerpt from an aminophylline guideline to help you.

NHS trust	Actual body weight: _____ kg	
Aminophylline infusion proforma	Aminophylline does not distribute into fatty tissue. Ideal body weight needs to be used for obese patients **Male: 50 kg + 2.3 kg for every inch over 5 ft** **Female: 45.5 kg + 2.3 kg for every inch over 5 ft**	
Intravenous loading dose = 5 mg/kg over 20 minutes		
Intravenous maintenance dose As continuous infusion Rates in mL/hr	Elderly/heart failure	0.3 mg/kg/hr
	Non-smoking adult	0.5 mg/kg/hr
	Smoking adult	0.7 mg/kg/hr

25   Jasmeet is an 8-year-old girl who has been admitted to the children's A & E with a severe asthma attack that has not responded to oxygen and nebulisers. When taking her history, you find that Jasmeet was already taking *Slo-Phyllin®* (theophylline) modified-release capsules 120 mg BD alongside inhalers, montelukast, and antihistamines. You also find that she weighs 24.6 kg. The medical team want to escalate her treatment and decide to initiate an aminophylline infusion. Jasmeet responds to the initial loading dose of aminophylline, but the medical team ask for your support with administering the maintenance infusion.

Given that the nursing staff will dilute one aminophylline 25 mg/mL vial to 250 mL in 0.9% sodium chloride, what rate should the infusion pump be set to initially? Give your answer to one decimal place.

You may use the SPC for aminophylline hydrate 25 mg/mL solution for injection to help you: https://www.medicines.org.uk/emc/product/6560/smpc

26   Mrs G comes to see you about losing weight and would like to try orlistat. During the consultation you find that Mrs G is 5 feet 1 inches tall and weighs 14 stones and 3 pounds.

What is Mrs G's body mass index expressed as a whole number? You may use the Approximate Conversions and Units page from the BNF to help you.

27   Mrs A has been admitted to your emergency department with suspected digoxin toxicity. After taking blood tests, her serum digoxin level is found to be 4.6 micrograms/L and the medical team want to initiate *DigiFab®*. Her weight on admission was 62.8 kg.

How many vials of *DigiFab®* should be supplied to treat Mrs A? Give your answer to the nearest whole number.

You may use the SPC for *DigiFab®* to help you: https://bit.ly/2tjxt18

28   Mr P, who weighs 78.3 kg, requires an intravenous infusion of dopamine hydrochloride, which has been prescribed at a rate of 3 micrograms/kg/minute. The nurses have infusion bags of 160 mg dopamine in 100 mL of glucose 5%.

At what rate should the infusion pump be set? Give your answer to one decimal place.

29   You are asked to make a chlorhexidine solution for the disinfection of wounds and burns.

What strength of chlorhexidine solution (mg/mL) do you need to prepare so that when 5 mL is diluted to 100 mL it gives a final concentration of 0.05% (w/v)? Give your answer to the nearest whole number.

30 You have received a prescription for 5% salicylic acid cream, which is not available in your pharmacy. You have a stock of the 2% cream and salicylic acid powder.
What weight of salicylic acid powder must you add to 100 g of 2% (w/w) salicylic acid cream to produce a cream of 5% (w/w)? Give your answer to three decimal places.

31 One of the nurses calls you from the neonatal intensive care unit regarding starter parenteral nutrition for one of her patients. Earlier in the day your pharmacy department supplied the ward with a 50 mL vial of glucose 50% and a 500 mL bag of glucose 20%. The nurse needs to make up a 50 mL syringe containing 37.5% glucose. What volume of glucose 50% will the nurse need to use? Give your answer to one decimal place.

32 Mr E was admitted to hospital with atrial fibrillation that required rapid correction with intravenous digoxin. On medical review he has responded well to the intravenous loading dose of 750 micrograms digoxin and the medical team want to place him on long term oral therapy aiming for a serum digoxin of 2.0 micrograms/L (acceptable range of 1.5–2.0 micrograms/L). You glean the following information from his notes:

Weight: 75 kg	**Height:** 6′ 0″	**Age:** 74 years
HR: 81 bpm	**BP:** 143/95	**Temp:** 37°C
Creatinine: 153 µmol/L	**K⁺:** 3.4 mmol/L	**Urea:** 6.1 mmol/L

Calculate the daily dose that Mr E should initially be prescribed. Give your answer to the nearest whole tablet.
You may use the SPC for digoxin tablets to help you: https://www.medicines.org.uk/emc/product/5464/smpc

33 Mrs C attends your respiratory clinic for a review of her COPD, which seems to have worsened over the past 6 months. She is currently taking salbutamol PRN and you are considering stepping up her treatment. In order to prescribe the optimal therapy, you decide to measure her FEV1, which you find to be 1.29 L/s.
Calculate Mrs C's FEV1 as a percentage of her predicted normal (2.10 L/s). Give your answer to the nearest whole number.

34 Miss H is one of your cystic fibrosis patients who presents with an outpatient prescription for piperacillin-tazobactam 4.5 g vials to be reconstituted with 0.9% sodium chloride, administered three times a day for 28 days. The prescription also calls for 10 mL sodium chloride 0.9% to be used to flush the PICC line before and after each dose of piperacillin-tazobactam.

How many 10 mL ampoules of sodium chloride 0.9% need to be dispensed? Round up your answer to the nearest 5 ampoules.

You may use the SPC for piperacillin 4g/ tazobactam 500 mg powder for solution for infusion vials to help you: https://www.medicines.org.uk/emc/product/8771

35 Mrs Q is 28 weeks pregnant and has been diagnosed with anaemia from iron deficiency. A trial with oral ferrous gluconate has failed to produce a clinically relevant response and the obstetric team now want to trial her on intravenous *Venofer*®. Mrs Q's notes contain the following information:

Age: 23 years

Height: 5′ 3″

Weight before pregnancy: 54 kg

Gestation: 28 weeks

Iron: 4.2 micromol/L

Haemoglobin: 8.6 g/dL

BP: 134/91 mmHg

Calculate the total dose of *Venofer*® Mrs Q will need to be given over the course of her treatment. Give your answer to the nearest whole number.

You may use the SPC for *Venofer*® to help you: https://www.medicines.org.uk/emc/product/5911

36 Mr S has been diagnosed with invasive group A streptococcal infection and the microbiologist has advised commencing benzylpenicillin at a dose of 1.2 g IV every four hours, given in 100 mL glucose 5%, infused over 60 minutes. His medical team are concerned about the sodium content of this product and ask you to calculate how much sodium the patient will receive.

How many millimoles of sodium will Mr S receive every 24 hours on this regimen? Give your answer to one decimal place.
You may use the SPC for benzylpenicillin to help you: www.medicines.org.uk/emc/medicine/32345

37   Mrs U is required to take co-trimoxazole for prophylaxis against spontaneous bacterial peritonitis at a dose of 960 mg each morning. Your pharmacy only stocks the 480 mg strength of co-trimoxazole. How many 480 mg co-trimoxazole tablets are required to cover a 4-week period? Give your answer to the nearest whole number.

38   Mr Y is taking warfarin for a prosthetic valve and has just been to the anticoagulation clinic to get his INR checked. He presents you with his yellow book which advises Mr Y to take 2 mg every day except Saturday and Sunday when he will take 1 mg.
How many packs of 28 warfarin 1 mg tablets do you need to supply to ensure Mr Y has enough for 4 weeks' treatment? Give your answer to the nearest whole number.

39   Leslie is a patient on your paediatric ward suffering from hypocalcaemia. On the ward round the consultant paediatrician would like to give Leslie an infusion containing 9.5 mmol of calcium over 8 hours and asks you to support the nurses to make up an appropriate IV infusion. You find the following molecular masses for compounds commonly used to make up intravenous infusions including parenteral nutrition.

Formula	g/mol
$CaCl_2$	110.88
$CaCl_2 \cdot 2H_2O$	147.01
KCl	74.55
$MgCl_2$	95.21
NaCl	58.44

How many millilitres of calcium chloride dihydrate solution 13.4% w/v should be used in this infusion? Give your answer to the nearest 0.1 mL.

40   You are working in a specialist manufacturing unit and are asked about making intrathecal injections of 5 mg in 3 mL amphotericin soluble. You know the product will need to be isotonic with the CSF, of which you find the average freezing point to be -0.5770°C.

From your research you learn you may need to add sodium chloride to the formulation to make it isotonic. You find the freezing point depression value of a 1% sodium chloride solution to be 0.5760°C and find the freezing point depression value of a 1% solution of soluble amphotericin to be 0.1242°C.

Formula for isotonic solutions:

$$W = \frac{f - a}{b}$$

W is the amount (% w/v) of adjusting compound to be added
f is the freezing point depression of the target body fluid
a is the freezing point depression of the drug solution(s)
b is the freezing point depression of a 1% solution of adjusting compound

Calculate what mass of sodium chloride must be included in a 3 mL injection to ensure it is isotonic. Give your answer to two decimal places.

41 Miss Z is going travelling and her GP calls you to discuss malaria prophylaxis as she will be visiting Niger. Miss Z will arrive in the capital city of Niamey, where she will stay for 1 week, before heading to visit family in Agadez for 5 weeks, then returning to the UK. You confirm that it will be unlikely for Miss Z to avoid exposure to the sun, so you suggest that the GP prescribes *Malarone*® (atovaquone/proguanil) tablets once daily.
How many tablets of *Malarone*® should be prescribed for Miss Z to give maximum protection? Give your answer to the nearest whole number.
You may use the NaTHNaC Travel Health Pro website for Niger to help you: https://travelhealthpro.org.uk/country/164/niger

42 Juliet is a 7-year-old girl, weighing 18.4 kg, on your paediatric intensive care unit and the medical team want to prescribe intravenous paracetamol every 6 hours for her.
How much paracetamol should be prescribed for each dose? Give your answer to the nearest 5 mg.
You may use the paracetamol monograph in the BNFC to help you.

43 Neil is a 4-year-old boy who has suspected chicken pox and also has a fever.
What volume of paracetamol 120 mg/5 mL oral solution should be given for each dose? Give your answer to the nearest whole number. You may use the paracetamol monograph in the BNFC to help you.

44 Mr H comes into your pharmacy with a prescription for flucloxacillin to treat his folliculitis. He has been prescribed flucloxacillin 500 mg every 6 hours, on an empty stomach, for 6 weeks until his next outpatient appointment.
How many flucloxacillin 500 mg capsules do you need to dispense to complete the course? Give your answer to the nearest whole number.

45 Mrs K has undergone an emergency splenectomy after being involved in a road traffic accident. To protect her against pneumococcal infections, she is due to be started on phenoxymethylpenicillin 250 mg twice daily for the next 2 years. You are processing her discharge letter and are notified that there are no 250 mg tablets in stock.
How many phenoxymethylpenicillin 125 mg tablets should be supplied to cover a 28-day period? Give your answer to the nearest whole number.

46 Mrs T has been diagnosed with infective endocarditis, caused by *Staphylococcus aureus*. She is now well enough to be discharged home, so the infectious diseases team have changed her IV vancomycin twice daily to IV teicoplanin, for three loading doses, then once daily maintenance doses to complete 4 weeks' treatment. Mrs T weighs 100 kg but her creatinine clearance is only 23.5 mL/min. How many vials of teicoplanin 400 mg solution for injection need to be supplied to cover the treatment? Give your answer to the nearest whole number.
You may use the SPC for teicoplanin 400 mg vials to help you: https://www.medicines.org.uk/emc/product/2927/smpc

47 You a reviewing a placebo-controlled clinical trial for a new statin for the primary prevention of stroke in patients with high cholesterol. Each trial arm contains 350 adults. 23 strokes were identified in the placebo arm, whereas 20 strokes were identified in the treatment arm.
Calculate the number needed to treat (NNT) for this trial.
You may use the BMJ Best Practice guide on 'How to calculate risk' to help you: https://bestpractice.bmj.com/info/toolkit/learn-ebm/how-to-calculate-risk/

48 You a reviewing a placebo-controlled clinical trial investigating adalimumab for treatment of hidradenitis suppurativa. The control arm contained 163 participants, of which 27.6% achieved clinical improvement during the follow-up period. The treatment arm contained 163 participants, of which 58.9% achieved clinical improvement during the follow-up period.

Calculate the absolute risk reduction (ARR) for adalimumab for the treatment of hidradenitis suppurativa. Give your answer to one decimal place.

You may use the BMJ Best Practice guide on 'How to calculate risk' to help you: https://bestpractice.bmj.com/info/toolkit/learn-ebm/how-to-calculate-risk/

49 You are reviewing a population cohort study investigating the ability of low-dose aspirin to prevent cancer over a 10-year period. The results found that 70,755 out of 408,339 people who did not take aspirin developed cancer, whereas 26,929 out of 204,170 people who were taking aspirin did develop cancer.

Calculate the relative risk reduction (RRR) for low-dose aspirin for the development of cancer over a 10-year period. Give your answer to one decimal place.

You may use the BMJ Best Practice guide on 'How to calculate risk' to help you: https://bestpractice.bmj.com/info/toolkit/learn-ebm/how-to-calculate-risk/

50 Jessica, a 3-year-old girl, has been admitted to your children's high dependency unit with suspected pesticide poisoning. The medical team want to give a loading dose of pralidoxime chloride, followed by a continuous infusion for a further 24 hours to counteract organophosphates. On admission Jessica was found to weigh 13.4 kg and was 87 cm tall.

How many vials of pralidoxime chloride should be supplied to cover this treatment? Give your answer to the nearest whole number.

You may use the pralidoxime chloride monograph in the BNFC to help you.

51 Miss U has been admitted to your emergency department with paracetamol overdose. For the first acetylcysteine infusion the medical team has prescribed a dose of 9690 mg acetylcysteine in glucose 5%. Calculate the rate at which the infusion pump should be set. Give your answer to two decimal places.

You may use the Emergency treatment of poisoning section in the BNF to help you.

52 Mr W is on your acute medical ward and the medical team want him to be given 1 litre of Hartmann's solution (potassium chloride with calcium chloride, sodium chloride and sodium lactate) to be infused over 6 hours. The nurse asks for your advice as there are no infusion pumps available and she will need to estimate the rate by the number of drops per minute.
Calculate the number of drops per minute. Give your answer as a whole number.

53 You are working as a biologics pharmacist and are tasked with reviewing patients on adalimumab and considering them for a switch away from *Humira*®, which costs £704.28 for two 40 mg prefilled pens, to the biosimilar product *Amgevita*®, which costs £633.60 for two 40 mg prefilled pens. You are focusing on the 102 people in your service who are using *Humira*® for the treatment of psoriatic arthritis, for which the dose is 40 mg every 2 weeks.
Assuming no overheads, other charges, or discounts, how much money can be saved per patient per 52 weeks once they have been switched to *Amgevita*®? Give your answer to the nearest pounds and pence.

54 Mrs C has been diagnosed with staphylococcal colonisation of her central venous catheter, which the medical team want to salvage with vancomycin line locks.
What volume of vancomycin 50 mg/mL solution for infusion do you need to use, so that when diluted to a final volume of 3 mL with 0.9% sodium chloride, the resultant vancomycin concentration is 10 mg/mL? Give your answer to one decimal place.

55 Mrs R has been admitted to your hospital with pyelonephritis, which has led to sepsis. The microbiology team want to give Mrs R a stat dose of IV ceftriaxone as an additional antimicrobial to manage her condition. The microbiology team want to achieve peak serum concentrations at least ten times greater than the break point of 2 mg/L.
What is the minimum peak serum concentration that is likely to be achieved with a 1 g dose of IV ceftriaxone? Give your answer to one decimal place.
You may use the SPC for ceftriaxone 1g powder for solution for injection to help you: https://www.medicines.org.uk/emc/product/1361/smp

56 Immediately after giving Mrs R a stat dose of 1 g IV ceftriaxone, a blood sample is taken to determine the serum concentration of ceftriaxone achieved. The laboratory reports a serum concentration of 106.8 mg/L. Given that ceftriaxone is a time-dependant antibacterial

agent, and the microbiology team want to achieve serum concentrations above the break point of 2 mg/L, you are asked to estimate what the serum concentration will be after 24 hours.

Estimate the serum concentration of ceftriaxone at 24 hours. Give your answer to one decimal place.

You may use the SPC for ceftriaxone 1g powder for solution for injection to help you: https://www.medicines.org.uk/emc/product/1361/smp

57 Mr J has been admitted to your ITU with suspected toxic epidermal necrolysis and the ITU team would like to commence an infusion of immunoglobulins. Mr J is 6 feet 1 inch tall and weighs 143.6 kg, so you remind the team that immunoglobulins should be dosed by a different, calculated, dose-determining weight in patients who are obese.

What weight should be used to determine the dose of immunoglobulin? Give your answer to the nearest whole number.

You may use the Department of Health's 'Clinical guidelines for immunoglobulin use' to help you: https://assets.publishing.service.gov.uk/government/uploads/system/uploads/attachment_data/file/216671/dh_131107.pdf

58 You are called out of hours to support with obtaining and administering intravenous immunoglobulins for a new born baby with haemolytic disease. The baby, Maaz, has a healthy weight of 4.2 kg and no other illness of note.

What dose of intravenous immunoglobulin should be prescribed for this patient? Give your answer to the nearest gram.

You may use the Department of Health's 'Clinical guidelines for immunoglobulin use' to help you: https://assets.publishing.service.gov.uk/government/uploads/system/uploads/attachment_data/file/216671/dh_131107.pdf

59 You are a commissioning pharmacist investigating potential cost savings that can be achieved through simple product switches. You are proposing that the 3256 patients currently prescribed omeprazole 20 mg once daily as dispersible tablets should be switched to lansoprazole 15 mg dispersible tablets once daily. The average price of a box of 28 omeprazole 20 mg dispersible tablets is £13.92, whereas the average price of a box of 28 lansoprazole 15 mg dispersible tablets is £2.99.

Assuming whole packs are dispensed and claimed, calculate the maximum annual cost saving for the CCG if this switch is performed. Give your answer to the nearest whole pound.

60   You are working in a HIV clinic and have recently been asked to find cost savings within the drug budget. Currently, your clinic dispenses *Truvada*® (emtricitabine 200 mg/ tenofovir 245 mg) to 235 of its clients with HIV. One 30-day pack of *Truvada*® costs £355.73 and your clinic supplies HIV medicines in 6-monthly instalments. However, a 30-pack of the generic emtricitabine 200 mg/ tenofovir 245 mg tablets can now be obtained for as little as £106.72.
Assuming that whole packs are dispensed, calculate the maximum saving that can be achieved over each 6-month period once all patients have been switched from *Truvada*® to the generic product. Give your answer to the nearest whole pound.

61   Mr U, who weighs 49.5 kg, has been diagnosed with cutaneous leishmaniasis and is prescribed IV pentamidine for treatment.
How many vials of pentamidine isethionate need to be supplied to cover the whole course?
You may use the SPC for *Pentacarinat*® powder for solution for injection to help you: https://www.medicines.org.uk/emc/product/977/smpc

62   Jakob is a 6-year-old boy who weighs 18.7 kg and has been diagnosed with a severe infection, for which the microbiologists have recommended IV fosfomycin at a dose of 100 mg/kg TDS. You have supplied enough of the fosfomycin 2 g vials to cover the entire treatment course.
What volume of the reconstituted fosfomycin vials should be drawn up for each dose? Give your answer to one decimal place.
You may use the SPC for *Fomicyt*® powder for solution for injection to help you: https://bit.ly/3aepcMm

63   Mrs V has been diagnosed with *Pneumocystis jirovecii (Pneumocystis carinii)* pneumonia and has been recommended co-trimoxazole tablets to be taken at an equal dose three times a day for the next 3 weeks. You find that Mrs V is 79 years old and weighs 57.6 kg.
How many co-trimoxazole 480 mg tablets should be dispensed to fulfil the treatment? Give your answer to the nearest whole number.
You may use the co-trimoxazole monograph in the BNF to help you.

64   Promise is a 6-year-old girl with pulmonary hypertension for which she is taking two sildenafil 10 mg tablets three times a day. She now needs to have her medicines administered through a temporary nasogastric feeding tube, so you recommend switching the sildenafil tablets to the oral suspension.

How many bottles of sildenafil oral suspension do you need to supply to cover a 4-week period? Give your answer to the nearest whole number.

You may use the sildenafil monograph in the BNFC to help you.

65   Mr Q has been admitted to your hospital with a severe flare of his Raynaud's. When undertaking his drug history, you find that he weighs 78.6 kg, smoked about 10 cigarettes per day, and was only taking simvastatin 20 mg at night before admission. The medical team want to trial Mr Q on an infusion of iloprost at the recommended dose of 0.5 nanogram/kg/minute for 30 minutes, during which time they will review his response and tolerance before deciding whether to continue.

The nurse has made up an infusion of 10 micrograms iloprost in 50 mL sodium chloride 0.9%.

At what rate should this infusion be given? Give your answer to one decimal place.

66   Mr A was admitted to your assessment unit due to alcohol withdrawal and was placed on a diazepam weaning regimen, starting at 10 mg QDS. He is now on day three of the weaning regimen and is due to go home at lunch time. Your hospital's diazepam weaning regimen is as follows:

Time	Day 1	Day 2	Day 3	Day 4	Day 5	Day 6	Day 7
08:00	10 mg	10 mg	10 mg	5 mg	5 mg		STOP
12:00	10 mg						
18:00	10 mg	10 mg	5 mg	5 mg			
22:00	10 mg	10 mg	10 mg	5 mg	5 mg	5 mg	

How many diazepam 5 mg tablets do you need to supply for the remainder of the weaning regimen? Give your answer to the nearest whole number.

67   You are developing a new formulation that requires glycerol to be used as an excipient. Your next batch of product will require 320 mL of glycerol to be added. However, glycerol is difficult to measure accurately by volume so you will need to add the respective mass of glycerol to your formulation during processing.

Given that the density of glycerol is 1.25 g/mL, what mass of glycerol will you need? Give your answer to the nearest whole number.

68   You are working in a specials manufacturing unit and are upscaling one of the otic formulations. The master formula requires 32% v/v arachis oil and you are planning to make a batch of 10 L of product. Due to the properties of arachis oil, and the equipment available, you will need to measure the mass of arachis oil, rather than the volume. Given that the density of arachis oil is 0.917 g/mL, what mass of arachis oil is required for this batch? Give your answer to one decimal place.

69   Ronan is a 3-year-old boy on your paediatric assessment unit who has been found to have low potassium levels. The paediatricians have prescribed *Kay-Cee-L*® (potassium chloride 75 mg/mL) at a dose of 30 mmol per day in two divided doses.
      What volume of *Kay-Cee-L*® syrup should be given to Ronan for each dose? Give your answer to the nearest whole millilitre.
      You may use the periodic table of elements to help you: https://www.ptable.com/

70   Miss W presents to your pharmacy with a prescription for ceftazidime 5% eye drops, two to three drops into the right eye TDS for 7 days. How many bottles containing 5 mL of ceftazidime 5% eye drops do you need to supply? Give your answer to the nearest whole number.

71   Mr Z is receiving intravenous maintenance fluids as he is not eating or drinking very well. The medical team have prescribed a 500 mL bag containing potassium chloride 0.15%, glucose 4% and sodium chloride 0.18% to be run over 4 hours. You want to check how much energy Mr Z is receiving throughout the day.
      How much glucose will Mr Z receive from this infusion? Give your answer to the nearest whole number.

72   Miss K has been admitted to your emergency department with a severe exacerbation of her asthma, but her breathing has not responded to initial bronchodilator treatment. The medical team has prescribed 2 g of magnesium chloride to be given by intravenous infusion over 20 minutes.
      What volume of magnesium chloride 50% (2 mmol/mL) solution for injection should be added to the infusion bag? Give your answer to the nearest whole number.

73   Mrs N is being treated for non-falciparum malaria with chloroquine oral syrup. The infectious diseases team has prescribed a dose of 620 mg STAT followed by doses of 310 mg after 6 hours, then daily for a further 2 days.

What volume of chloroquine 80 mg/5 mL syrup is required to give the first dose of 620 mg? Give your answer to the nearest whole number. You may use the chloroquine monograph in the BNF to help you.

74 Mrs H has been prescribed potassium permanganate leg soaks, which is achieved by soaking dressings in a 1 in 10000 solution of potassium permanganate then applying to the legs. Your pharmacy stocks *Permitabs*®, which contain 400 mg of potassium permanganate per tablet.
    In what volume of water should one *Permitabs*® be dissolved in to achieve the desired solution? Give your answer to the nearest whole number.

75 Richard is 14 years old and has been diagnosed with allergic rhinitis. His GP has prescribed fluticasone nasal spray 100 mcg into each nostril twice daily.
    How many days treatment will two 50 microgram/dose nasal sprays, each containing 150 doses, provide? Give your answer to one decimal place.

76 You are working in an allergy clinic and need to prepare a series of diluted suspensions of amphotericin B for an oral allergy challenge. You have access to a 100 mg/mL suspension of amphotericin B available, which you decide to dilute 1 in 10 for eight serial dilutions. Once prepared, the patient will take 5 mL of each suspension, starting from weakest, every 20 minutes under monitoring.
    What concentration of amphotericin B will be in the 8th serial dilution of the suspension? Give your answer to the nearest whole number.

77 Mr S is taking levothyroxine tablets every morning for hypothyroidism at a dose of 25 mcg or 50 mcg on alternate days. For a number of years Mr S has only been using the 25 mcg tablets to achieve both doses.
    How many 25 mcg tablets must be dispensed to cover a typical 28-day period? Give your answer to the nearest whole number.

78 Mrs J is taking methotrexate for remission of Crohn's disease. She presents to your pharmacy with a prescription for methotrexate 20 mg weekly, on Sundays, for 12 weeks. In line with national standards, you only dispense 2.5 mg methotrexate tablets.
    How many methotrexate 2.5 mg tablets need to be dispensed? Give your answer to the nearest whole number.

79 Mr B has been suffering from ulcerative colitis for a number of years and his gastroenterologist wants to commence him on golimumab.

You receive a prescription for golimumab 200 mg initially, followed by 100 mg after 2 weeks, then 100 mg every 4 weeks to complete a total of 18 weeks treatment.

How many golimumab 100 mg prefilled pens need to be supplied in total? Give your answer to the nearest whole number.

80   Mr F is a patient on your HDU whose serum creatinine is 137 μmol/L and his eGFR has been reported at 31 mL/min/1.73m² through the laboratory result system. You note he is 83 years old and only weighs 57.6 kg.

Estimate Mr F's renal function using the Cockcroft and Gault formula. Give your answer to one decimal place.

You may use the Prescribing in renal impairment section in the BNF to help you.

81   You are working as a community pharmacist and Mrs A, a 42-year-old lady, comes into your pharmacy with her repeat prescription for fluoxetine 10 mg capsules, two to be taken once daily for 28 days. There are no fluoxetine 10 mg capsules available from the suppliers, and you are unable to obtain the 10 mg tablets. After a discussion with the patient, she agrees to take the oral solution, which you can supply under a serious shortage protocol.

What volume of fluoxetine oral solution does Mrs A require? Give your answer to the nearest whole number.

You may use the serious shortage protocol for fluoxetine 10 mg capsules (SSP01 October 2019) to help you: https://www.nhsbsa.nhs .uk/sites/default/files/2019-10/SSP%20Fluoxetine%2010mg%20 capsules_0.pdf

82   Tabitha is a 6-year-old girl on your paediatric surgery ward who has been diagnosed with a joint infection. The paediatricians would like to commence vancomycin until she is well enough to take oral medicines. Tabitha weighs 18.3 kg, is 1.12 m tall, and her serum creatinine is 47 micromol/L.

Estimate Tabitha's glomerular filtration rate to determine her renal function. Give your answer to one decimal place.

You may use the SPC for vancomycin to help you: https://www .medicines.org.uk/emc/product/649/smpc

83   Mr K has been diagnosed with his third episode of *Clostridioides difficile* diarrhoea. The specialist nurse has prescribed the following vancomycin weaned-pulsed regimen to treat Mr K's current infection and prevent further infections.

> **Mr K**
> **NHS: 999 999**
>
> Vancomycin capsules 125 mg QDS for 10 days, then 125 mg TDS for one week, then 125 mg BD for one week, then 125 mg OD for one week, then 125 mg every other day for 3 doses, then 125 mg every 72-hours for 2 doses.
>
> Edwards
> C.difficile specialist nurse
> 1/2/2020

How many vancomycin 125 mg capsules do you need to supply to complete the prescribed course? Give your answer to the nearest whole number.

84   Imran is an 8-year-old boy who has been diagnosed with invasive aspergillosis, which is to be treated with IV caspofungin. The paediatricians ask for your help in calculating the loading dose for Imran. Looking at his notes you find he is 24.1 kg in weight and 126.9 cm tall.

Calculate the loading dose of caspofungin required for Imran. Give your answer to the nearest 5 mg.

You may use the SPC for caspofungin vials to help you: https://www .medicines.org.uk/emc/product/2226/smpc

85   Mrs S is suffering from atrial fibrillation and after a loading dose of digoxin her consultant wants to trial a daily maintenance dose of intravenous digoxin because she is too unwell to swallow. The consultant would like to aim for a serum digoxin concentration of 2.0 micrograms/L (acceptable range of 1.5–2.0 micrograms/L).

Estimate the daily dose that Mrs S should be prescribed. Give your answer to the nearest 5 mcg.

> The following information is available in her medical notes:
>
> | | | |
> |---|---|---|
> | **Weight:** 50.1 kg | **Height:** 5′ 2″ | **Age:** 68 years |
> | **HR:** 86 bpm | **BP:** 136/84 | **Temp:** 37.2°C |
> | **Creatinine:** 136 µmol/L | **K⁺:** 4.3 mmol/L | **Urea:** 3.9 mmol/L |
> | **Creatinine clearance = 27.6 mL/min** | | **NT-ProBNP:** 206 pg/mL |

You can utilise the following digoxin pharmacokinetic formulae:

$$C_{pss} = \frac{(F \times D)}{(DigCl \times t)}$$

Non-heart failure DigCl (L/hr) = [0.06 × creatinine clearance (mL/min)] + [0.05 × IBW (kg)

Heart failure DigCl (L/hr) = [0.053 × creatinine clearance (mL/min)] + [0.02 × IBW (kg)]

Male IBW = 50 kg + 2.3 kg for every inch over 5ft

Female IBW = 45.5 kg + 2.3 kg for every inch over 5ft

86 One of your patients, Mr N, has been prescribed phenobarbital 680 mg by intravenous injection for the management of status epilepticus.

What is the shortest amount of time over which the infusion can be given? Give your answer to the nearest whole minute.

You may use the phenobarbital monograph in the BNF to help you.

87 Mr T is an 81-year-old man who weighs 82.6 kg who has been admitted to your coronary care unit with suspected ST-elevated myocardial infarction. He is not suitable for percutaneous coronary intervention, but the medical team would like to immediately start subcutaneous enoxaparin every 12 hours.

What dose of subcutaneous enoxaparin should be prescribed? Give your answer to the nearest whole milligram.

You may use the enoxaparin monograph in the BNF to help you.

88 You are having a discussion with Mrs V about her medicines and find out that she has not been taking her iron supplements because she must take so many and they are giving her constipation. She should be taking two ferrous gluconate 300 mg tablets three times a day. You suggest that a different iron-containing tablet, ferrous fumarate, may alleviate this problem.

How many ferrous fumarate 200 mg tablets should Mrs V take each day?

89 Your central hospital procurement service stocks 8 in 10 acetic acid solution, available in 500 mL bottles, which is supplied to your hospital's theatres. Whilst reviewing the theatre procedures,

the department practitioners ask you to check the instructions for diluting this stock solution.

What volume of this stock solution is required so that when it is diluted to 5 litres the final concentration is 3% w/v? Give your answer to one decimal place.

90   You are testing a batch of tablets for the content of heavy metals. You are utilising atomic absorption spectrometry to determine the concentration of lead (Pb) in the tablets, for which there is a limit of 10 ppm. Your test determines the concentration of lead in the tablets is 7.2 ng/g.

What is the concentration, in parts per million, of lead in this batch of tablets? Give your answer to two significant figures.

91   Alex is a 14-year-old patient on your teenager and young adult cystic fibrosis ward who has been admitted for a course of once daily intravenous amikacin. The post-dose peak amikacin level comes back from the lab as 32.3 mg/L. You advise the team that another dose should not be given unless the trough level is less than 5 mg/L. To enable you to model the amikacin pharmacokinetics in Alex, which usually has a terminal half-life of 2–3 hours, you ask for another amikacin level to be taken 6 hours after the dose was given.

Estimate what the highest amikacin concentration should be in the level taken at 6 hours. Give your answer to one decimal place.

92   Mrs D is approaching the end of her life and is struggling to swallow food and medicines. The nursing team feel that Mrs D's chronic pain, secondary to cancer, would be better managed using a syringe driver. When looking at her chart you find Mrs D has been taking one morphine sulfate 60 mg modified-release capsule and one morphine sulfate 30 mg modified-release capsule twice daily for the past 6 months.

How much morphine sulfate needs to be made up in the syringe driver to deliver the appropriate dose over 24 hours? Give your answer to the nearest whole number.

You may use the Prescribing in palliative care section in the BNF to help you.

93   You are working in a hospital and have been asked to review Mr L, who is with you for end of life care due to progressive osteosarcoma. The nurses are concerned that the *OxyNorm*® oral liquid is not adequately relieving his breakthrough pain. Looking at his prescriptions you notice that the dose of oxycodone modified-release tablets was recently increased from 50 mg BD to 60 mg BD, but the dose of *OxyNorm*® had not been altered.

What is the minimum volume of *OxyNorm*® (oxycodone 5 mg/5 mL) oral liquid that Mr L should be given for episodes of breakthrough pain? Give your answer to the nearest whole number.

You may use the Prescribing in palliative care section in the BNF to help you.

94   Mr C is an 81-year-old man on your medical admissions unit who is unable to swallow safely. Before admission, Mr C was taking one co-careldopa 50 mg/200 mg modified-release tablet at 10pm, and one co-careldopa 12.5 mg/50 mg tablet at 7am, 10am, 2pm and 6pm. The medical team ask for your help in converting this medicine to the appropriate rotigotine patch.

What total strength of rotigotine patch(es) should be prescribed? Give your answer to the nearest whole number.

You may use the Emergency management of patient's with Parkinson's guide from Parkinson's UK to help you: https://www.parkinsons.org.uk/sites/default/files/2017-12/pk0135_emergencymanagement.pdf

95   Ijeoma is a 16-year-old girl on the intensive care unit who requires sedation during ventilation. The anaesthetists have prescribed a dose of propofol of 0.3 mg/kg/hour initially, which they will review in line with Ijeoma's response. You find that Ijeoma weighed 49.8 kg on admission to your intensive care unit. The unit stocks propofol 1% emulsion for intravenous infusion.

At what rate should the propofol infusion be given? Give your answer to two decimal places.

96   You are developing a formula of a new oral solution and want to mask the flavour of the drug molecule using clove oil. In your master formula you decide to replace 75 mL of the potable water with clove oil but want to measure it directly by weight as this will avoid any loss due to adherence to measuring cylinders.

Given that the specific gravity of clove oil is 1.04, what mass should be added to the formulation? Give your answer to the nearest whole number.

Formula for calculating specific gravity:

$$\text{Specific gravity} = \frac{\text{Weight of substance}}{\text{Weight of equal volume of water}}$$

97 You are working in a non-sterile manufacturing facility and receive an order for 500 mL of an extemporaneously prepared oral suspension containing capecitabine 500 mg/5 mL. You have access to the following master formula.

Capecitabine 500 mg/5 mL oral suspension

Formula:

    37 capecitabine 500 mg tablets

    92.5 mL Oral Plus

    92.5 mL Oral Sweet

Method:

    1) Crush capecitabine tablets in a mortar.

    2) Mix with Oral Plus.

    3) Add in Oral Sweet.

    4) Mix for 15 minutes until tablets fully disintegrated and dispersed.

How many capecitabine 500 mg tablets are required to make the required suspension? Give your answer to the nearest whole number.

98 You are working in a radiopharmacy suite and receive an order for a vial of technetium medronic acid 30 mCi, which will be used at 13:00 to perform a bone scan. The radiopharmacy technicians will need to prepare the product at 07:00 to allow for checking and transport. The half-life of Tc^{99m} is 6 hours and your radiopharmacy suite records radioactivity in the SI unit of becquerel (Bq).
What activity is required at the point of dispensing to ensure the correct radioactive dose is given? Give your answer to the nearest whole number.

Table of equivalents

1 Ci	3.7×10^4 MBq
1 mCi	37 MBq
1 Bq	2.7 10-11 Ci
1 MBq	2.7×10-5 Ci

99   Mrs A needs betamethasone 0.05% ointment to treat an inflamma-
     tory skin condition on both of her legs. The GP wants Mrs A to
     use the ointment twice a day for the next 2 weeks then return for a
     follow-up appointment. The GP asks for your advice on how much
     betamethasone 0.05% ointment to prescribe.
     Given that betamethasone 0.05% ointment is available in pack sizes
     of 30 g and 100 g, how much should be prescribed? Give your answer
     to the nearest whole number.
     You may use the Topical corticosteroids section in the BNF to help
     you.

100 You are presented with a prescription for Lassar's Paste to be applied
     to the affected area(s) twice daily, supply 100 g. You do not have this
     in stock but do have the constituent ingredients available. You plan
     to make a 3% excess to ensure the full amount can be dispensed to
     the patient.
     What mass of salicylic acid BP is required to prepare this product?
     Give your answer to the nearest whole number.
     You may use the zinc and salicylic acid paste BP (Lassar's Paste)
     monograph in the BNF to help you.

Single best answers

SECTION A

1 E

3 months use OTC. See patient information leaflet: https://www
.medicines.org.uk/emc/product/844/pil

2 A

A - correct, see PIL: https://www.medicines.org.uk/emc/files/pil.1317
.pdf; B - incorrect, treat all family members regardless of infective
state; C - not licensed OTC in pregnancy; D - incorrect, licensed in
ages 2+; E - incorrect, usually a one off stat dose.

3 D

A - incorrect because nil purulent discharge - usually yellow/sticky;
B - incorrect because usually bilateral; C - incorrect because usually
involves pain and photophobia; D - correct because usually unilateral, nil pain, self-limiting; E - incorrect because usually bilateral
with discharge.

4 B

A - active ingredient contains 60 mg per tablets; B - correct license, see
PIL: https://www.medicines.org.uk/emc/files/pil.6199.pdf; C - can
cause BG's to raise; D - can cause BP to rise; E - not for epistaxis.

5 A

Most likely haemorrhoids.

6 E

7 B
Gastric ulcer concerns - symptoms could be dangerous, patient needs urgent referral to A & E.

8 E
Ringworm management usually first line is to manage with an antifungal OTC.

9 A
Refer to GP - do not supply as patient has diabetes. See PIL: https://www.medicines.org.uk/emc/files/pil.296.pdf

10 A
Not licensed for supply in under 2 year olds: https://www.rpharms.com/resources/quick-reference-guides/chloramphenicol-05w-v-eye-drops-1w-v-ointment

11 B
See BNF, Appendix 1: Interactions, Fentanyl.

12 E
See BNF monograph for isotretinoin. A - patients are required to take contraception; B - monitoring needed for liver function tests; C - patients with a history of depression require close monitoring; D - causes decreased libido; E - correct.

13 A
See MEP, Professional and legal issues: Prescription-only medicines, Supplying oral retinoids and pregnancy prevention.

14 D
As per NICE: https://cks.nice.org.uk/lipid-modification-cvd-prevention#!scenario

15 D
See BNF monograph for risedronate sodium (alendronic acid not licensed in men).

ANSWERS

16 C

As per NICE: https://cks.nice.org.uk/atrial-fibrillation. Consider anticoagulation therapy if risk score 1 or above, can be warfarin or NOAC.

17 E

See BNF monograph for metronidazole.

18 C

https://about-cancer.cancerresearchuk.org/about-cancer/breast-cancer/getting-diagnosed/screening/breast-screening

19 C

Fluoxetine is associated with a lower risk of withdrawal symptoms if stopped abruptly due to longer half-life. See BNF monograph for fluoxetine.

20 E

See BNF monograph for mirtazapine.

21 D

See BNF monograph for minocycline.

22 E

Max dose in above 65 year olds is 20 mg daily, needs to reduce dose due to risk of QT prolongation. See alert: https://www.gov.uk/drug-safety-update/citalopram-and-escitalopram-qt-interval-prolongation

23 A

Both sertraline and naproxen can increase the risk of a bleed - consider adding in a PPI to protect lining of stomach; dose is correct for rheumatoid arthritis. See BNF, Appendix 1: Interactions, Sertraline.

24 D

All the above can increase weight gain (common side effect). Can refer to routine listing in BNF.

25 D

See BNF monograph for lithium carbonate.

26 B
See NHS: https://www.gloshospitals.nhs.uk/our-services/services-we
-offer/pathology/tests-and-investigations/digoxin/

27 A
See BNF monograph for prednisolone. Stopped long-term steroids
one year ago, consider a gradual reduction for this acute course to
prevent withdrawal.

28 D
https://www.nhs.uk/conditions/croup/. This is indicative of croup,
refer to A & E.

29 E
Likely otitis externa (swimmers ear): https://cks.nice.org.uk/otitis-
externa#!scenario:1

30 E
As per BNF monograph for allopurinol and SPC: https://www
.medicines.org.uk/emc/product/5693/smpc

31 D
See BNF monograph for aripiprazole and SPC: https://www
.medicines.org.uk/emc/product/3544/smpc

32 D
See BNF monograph for clozapine.

33 C
See BNF monograph for alendronic acid and BNF, Appendix 1:
Interactions, Alendronate.

34 E
Severe interaction, all others are potential considerations depending
on local guidance, patient's kidney function and past sensitivities to
microbe culture.

35 C
See BNF monograph for levothyroxine sodium.

36 C

See NHS: https://www.nhs.uk/conditions/cervical-screening/when-youll-be-invited/

37 C

A - can still prescribe cautiously in BMI >30; B - can still be issued as this is max recommended BP; C - avoid combined pill in migraine with aura; D - only relevant if patient started smoking; E - missed pill can be managed in the community with advice.

38 A

See BNF monograph for estradiol.

39 A

See BNF, Genito-urinary system, Contraception overview.

40 D

Max dose is 16 mg per day. See BNF monograph for loperamide hydrochloride.

41 B

See BNF monograph for medroxyprogesterone acetate.

42 E

A pharmacist or doctor can make the diagnosis, see RPS POM to P switch for sumatriptan.

43 C

Query impetigo, needs to be seen by GP: https://www.nhsinform.scot/illnesses-and-conditions/infections-and-poisoning/impetigo

44 C

See BNF monograph for metoclopramide hydrochloride.

45 D

See BNF monograph for empagliflozin.

46 A

See SPC: https://www.medicines.org.uk/emc/product/27/smpc

ANSWERS

47 E

See BNF, Respiratory system, Acute asthma overview.

48 E

See SPC: https://www.medicines.org.uk/emc/product/40/smpc

49 B

Lactulose can be supplied for this age, senna and bisacodyl cannot, no need to refer yet. See SPCs: https://www.medicines.org.uk/emc /product/5644/smpc, https://www.medicines.org.uk/emc/product/ 5525/smpc, https://www.medicines.org.uk/emc/product/8462/smpc

50 E

The first-line method is always to offer a copper intra-uterine device. See BNF, Genito-urinary system, Emergency contraception overview.

SECTION B

1 D

Enteric bacteria are documented as the most common causes of travellers' diarrhoea including several types of *Escherichia coli*. Also, *Campylobacter*, *Salmonella* and *Shigella* may cause travellers' diarrhoea. Travellers' diarrhoea is one of the most common illnesses in people who travel internationally and depending on destination affects 20–60% of the more than 800 million travellers each year. Source: https://www.bmj.com/content/353/bmj.i1937

2 C

All other factors are linked to travellers' diarrhoea apart from gender. Both genders are equally susceptible to traveller's diarrhoea. Source: https://www.bmj.com/content/353/bmj.i1937

3 C

Serum lipids (fasting values) should be checked before treatment, 1 month after the start of treatment, and subsequently at 3-monthly intervals unless more frequent monitoring is clinically indicated. Elevated serum lipid values usually return to normal on reduction of the dose or discontinuation of treatment and may also respond to dietary measures. Isotretinoin has been associated with an increase in plasma triglyceride levels. Isotretinoin should be discontinued if hypertriglyceridaemia cannot be controlled at an acceptable level or if symptoms of pancreatitis occur. Source: https://www.medicines .org.uk/emc/product/3870/smpc#UNDESIRABLE_EFFECTS

4 A

Patients prescribed alitretinoin must not donate blood during therapy and for 1 month after discontinuation due to the potential risk to the foetus of a pregnant transfusion recipient. Source: https://www.medicines.org.uk/emc/rmm/1513/Document

5 B

Most children get better within 3 days without antibiotics, however as symptoms persist in this child, antibiotic treatment is acceptable. The prescriber has issued a back-up (delayed) prescription in case symptoms worsen or don't improve within a

ANSWERS

specified time. The prescription may be given during the consultation (which may be a post-dated prescription) or left at an agreed location for collection at a later date. Source: https://www.nice.org.uk/guidance/ng91/documents/draft-guideline

6 E

A - Opportunity cost is defined as the benefit foregone when selecting one therapeutic alternative over the next best alternative; B - Cost benefit analysis(CBA) is a form of economic evaluation most useful for resource allocation investigation between government-financed activities and within the productive sectors; C - Cost-effectiveness analysis (CEA) is defined as an analytical technique intended for the systematic comparative evaluation of the overall cost and benefit generated by alternative therapeutic interventions for the management of a disease; D - Cost minimisation analysis (CMA) compares the cost of two similar interventions to ascertain which is less expensive; E - Cost utility analysis (CUA) is an economic analysis in which the incremental cost of a program from a particular point of view is compared to the incremental health improvement expressed in the unit of quality adjusted life years (QALYs). Source: https://www.sciencedirect.com/topics/nursing-and-health-professions/cost-utility-analysis

7 C

In patients with renal impairment avoid use of naproxen if eGFR less than $30\,mL/minute/1.73\,m^2$. See BNF monograph for naproxen.

8 D

Allopurinol is used as a prophylaxis for gout. The BNF cautions patients to ensure adequate fluid intake (2–3 L/day). Allopurinol should be withdrawn immediately when a skin rash or other evidence of sensitivity occurs as this could result in more serious hypersensitivity reactions (including Stevens-Johnson syndrome and toxic epidermal necrolysis) according to the SPC, Section 4.4 Special warnings and precautions for use. Source: https://www.medicines.org.uk/emc/product/5693/smpc#CLINICAL_PRECAUTIONS

9 E

Foods high in purine such as offal e.g. liver and kidneys, heart and sweetbreads should be avoided as can trigger acute gout attacks. Legumes such as baked beans, kidney beans, soya beans and peas etc. have moderate levels of purine, therefore should be eaten in moderation but is not necessary to totally eliminate. Foods low in purine content include dairy (milk, cheese, yoghurt, butter), eggs, bread and cereals (except wholegrain), pasta and noodles, and fruit and vegetables. See UK Gout Society for further dietary advice: http://www.ukgoutsociety.org/docs/goutsociety-allaboutgoutanddiet-0113.pdf

10 D

Infections are the most common complications seen in cancer patients and occur as a result of the underlying malignancy and of the various modalities used for treatment. Solid tumours are much more common than hematologic malignancies. The National Cancer Institute has defined solid tumours as non-cystic masses (either benign or malignant) including carcinomas, lymphomas and sarcomas. The vast majority will be solid tumours with cancers of the breast, lungs and bronchus, prostate, colon and rectum and urinary bladder being the most common. The most frequent cause of neutropenia is antineoplastic chemotherapy. Varying degrees of neutropenia also occur after radiation therapy. Source: https://www.ncbi.nlm.nih.gov/pmc/articles/PMC5336421/

ANSWERS

11 E

Oral vancomycin is recommended to treat confirmed severe cases of *C. difficile*. See NICE guidance: https://cks.nice.org.uk/diarrhoea-antibiotic-associated#!scenarioRecommendation:4

12 B

The trial did not include long-term safety and efficacy as was conducted in a 4-month window.

13 D

A type II error is a type of statistical error that occurs when the null hypothesis is false. For instance, when it is concluded that a treatment or intervention is not effective when it is. For this reason, it is also referred to as a false negative. Source: https://www.medicinenet.com/script/main/art.asp?articlekey=5876

14 D
    RRR (relative risk reduction) = (ARC* − ART*) / ARC
    (20 − 12) / 20 = (8 / 20) = 0.4 × 100 = 40%
    Source: https://bestpractice.bmj.com/info/us/toolkit/learn-ebm/how-to-calculate-risk/

15 A
    The patient does not want to undergo treatment therefore it goes against the principle of autonomy. The patient is a child but still has the right to autonomous decision making with regards to her own health and well-being. This ethos underpins patient-centred care.

16 B
    Insulin is safe to take during pregnancy to treat diabetes because insulin does not pass the placental barrier. When the patient plans to become pregnant and during pregnancy it is recommended that diabetes is not treated with metformin, but insulin be used to maintain blood glucose levels as close to normal as possible, to reduce the risk of malformations of the foetus. Beta-adrenoceptor blocking drugs (propranolol) are not teratogenic, however they do reduce placental perfusion, which may result in intra-uterine foetal death, immature and premature deliveries, therefore it should only be taken unless it is essential. Isotretinoin is highly teratogenic and therefore in pregnancy is an absolute contraindication. Women of childbearing potential have to use effective contraception during and up to one month after treatment. If pregnancy does occur in spite of these precautions during treatment with isotretinoin or in the month following, there is a great risk of very severe and serious malformation of the foetus. Use of ibuprofen during the third trimester is contraindicated as there is there is a risk of premature closure of the foetal ductus arteriosus with possible persistent pulmonary hypertension. The onset of labour may be delayed, and the duration increased with an increased bleeding tendency in both mother and child. Source: https://www.medicines.org.uk/emc/product/7886/smpc#PREGNANCY

17 A
    In patients over the age of 50 levothyroxine should be initiated in lower doses than that of younger patients. Source: https://www.ncbi.nlm.nih.gov/books/NBK279005/

18 D

Approximately 80% of acute pancreatitis is caused by gallstones (45%) and alcohol ingestion (35%). Other causes include some medicines such as thiazides, some antibiotics e.g. tetracycline, trimethoprim-sulfamethoxazole, medicines that suppress the immune system such as azathioprine, aminosalicylates, diuretics, valproate, etc. However, propranolol is not likely to cause pancreatitis. Very rarely, infections, trauma or surgery of the abdomen can cause pancreatitis. In about 10% of the cases, the cause is unknown (idiopathic). Source: https://my.clevelandclinic.org/health/diseases/17319-pancreatitis-acute--chronic-overview

19 C

Prophylactic enoxaparin is contraindicated following an acute stroke (for at least two months but varies according to hospital).

20 A

Intramuscular adrenaline must be administered in the first instance, then oxygen at the highest concentration possible. Following initial resuscitation give slow IM or IV chlorphenamine and slow IM or IV hydrocortisone (especially in people with asthma). Consider nebulised salbutamol or ipratropium if the person is wheezy (especially in people with known asthma). Source: https://cks.nice.org.uk/angio-oedema-and-anaphylaxis#!scenario:1

21 C

Hyperosmotic agents are used to treat corneal oedema to draw fluid away from the eye.

22 E

Nitrate tolerance development may be prevented by intermittent nitrate administration providing intervals with low plasma and tissue nitrate levels. Tolerance can occur regardless of age or route of administration.

23 A

The patient is suffering from a severe flare up of ulcerative colitis with more than 6 bowel motions per day and is hospitalised as a result, therefore in this case, IV steroids are required.

ANSWERS

24 B
Doxorubicin is a DNA binding drug which is absorbed locally, enters the cells and binds to their DNA, precipitating the death of the cell. Following this, the drug can then be re-released to further destroy healthy cells leading to deeper erosion of cells within the tissue. All of the other antineoplastics listed are non-DNA binding. Non-DNA binding drugs initiate cell death by mechanisms other than binding DNA and are eventually metabolised in the tissue and are more easily neutralised than the DNA binding vesicants. Extravasation and other injuries resulting from these agents generally remain localised and improve over time.

25 A
Degarelix is a gonadotrophin-releasing hormone (GnRH) blocker used to treat testicular cancer and is a type of hormonal therapy not immunotherapy. Source: https://www.cancerresearchuk.org/about-cancer/cancer-in-general/treatment/hormone-therapy/for-cancer

26 C
The SPC classifies side effects as: Very common ($\geq$1/10); common ($\geq$1/100 to <1/10); uncommon ($\geq$1/1,000 to <1/100); rare ($\geq$1/10,000 to <1/1,000); very rare (<1/10,000).

27 A
Buspirone may cause sleep disturbance but has not been linked with nightmares. A common side effect of propranolol, paroxetine and sertraline are nightmares. Nightmares and vivid dreams have also been reported with benzodiazepines. Zopiclone may cause nightmares but it is listed as uncommon in the SPC.

28 E
Although the patient has slightly elevated levels of potassium and urea, the high levels of creatinine indicate renal failure and must be prioritised. Ramipril is an ACE inhibitor and reduces the angiotensin II production necessary for preserving glomerular filtration when renal blood flow is reduced.

29 A
The symptoms the patient is presenting with are indicative of lithium toxicity. Additional symptoms include vomiting, diarrhoea, muscle

weakness, drowsiness and lack of coordination. Lithium toxicity is made worse by sodium depletion therefore concurrent use of thiazide diuretics should be avoided.

30 C

31 B
Intravenous is the only route vincristine should be administered. Vinka alkaloids must not be given intrathecally due to risk of death, or subcutaneously due to tissue necrosis.

32 E
Gynecomastia is the swelling of the breast tissue in boys or men, caused by an imbalance of the hormones oestrogen and testosterone. Spironolactone induces gynecomastia by blocking androgen production, blocking androgens from binding to their receptors, and by increasing both total and free oestrogen levels. Generally, the effects are reversible after discontinuation of the drug. Other drugs that can induce gynaecomastia include digoxin and centrally acting agents such as clonidine, methyldopa, reserpine and others. Source: https://www.ncbi.nlm.nih.gov/pmc/articles/PMC2719518/

33 A
Chlamydia is one of the most common sexually transmitted infections (STIs) in the UK. An annual chlamydia test is recommended for people under the age of 25 who are sexually active and each time the patient has a new sexual partner. In this case, symptoms indicate that the patient may have contracted chlamydia. However, it is important to note that many patients with chlamydia may not have any symptoms at all. Trichomoniasis is a STI caused by a parasite called *Trichomonas vaginalis* (TV), and while some symptoms are similar to chlamydial infection, patients with TV infection may also experience soreness and swelling and itching around the vagina and inner thighs. Source: https://cks.nice.org.uk/chlamydia-uncomplicated-genital#!diagnosisSub

34 B
Blood volume refers to the total amount of fluid circulating within the arteries, capillaries, veins, venules and chambers of the heart at any time. The amount of blood circulating within an individual depends

on their size and weight, but the average human adult has nearly 5 litres of circulating blood. Women tend to have a lower blood volume than men. However, a woman's blood volume increases by roughly 50% during pregnancy. Source: https://www.ncbi.nlm .nih.gov/books/NBK526077/

35 B
Two medicinal products containing the same active substance are considered bioequivalent if they are pharmaceutically equivalent or pharmaceutical alternatives and their bioavailabilities (rate and extent) after administration in the same molar dose lie within acceptable predefined limits. Source: https://www.ema .europa.eu/en/documents/scientific-guideline/guideline-investigation-bioequivalence-rev1_en.pdf

36 E
Community-acquired pneumonia (CAP) is defined as pneumonia that is acquired outside hospital. CAP can be caused by several different bacteria and viruses. *Streptococcus pneumoniae* is the commonest cause of CAP. *Streptococcus pneumoniae* is associated with the highest mortality rate in adults with community-acquired pneumonia. Parainfluenza virus causes croup in infants. *Pneumocystis jirovecii* is one of the most common causes of pneumonia in infants infected with HIV, responsible for at least one quarter of all pneumonia deaths in HIV-infected infants. Source: https://www .nice.org.uk/guidance/cg191/documents/pneumonia-final-scope2

37 E
Polycystic ovary syndrome (PCOS) is a heterogeneous endocrine disorder that appears to emerge at puberty. The clinical features may include hyperandrogenism (with clinical manifestations of oligomenorrhoea (absence of period), hirsutism, and acne), ovulation disorders and polycystic ovarian morphology. The clinical features vary widely, with symptoms of hyperandrogenism and severe menstrual disturbances at one end of the spectrum (previously known as Stein–Leventhal syndrome), and mild symptoms at the other. The symptoms that a woman with PCOS experiences may also vary over time. Source: https://cks.nice.org.uk/polycystic-ovary-syndrome#!backgroundSub

38 C
Metformin has been used in PCOS on the basis that it will reduce the effects of high serum insulin and androgen concentrations in patients. Although metformin is not licensed for the treatment of PCOS, the BNF has suggested a dosage regimen for off-label use. Metformin may reduce androgen levels by about 11% in women with PCOS compared with placebo. Source: https://cks.nice.org.uk/polycystic-ovary-syndrome#!scenario

39 A
Cervical cancer is not linked to polycystic ovary syndrome. However, insulin resistance is present in around 65–80% of women with PCOS. About 20–40% of obese women with PCOS have glucose intolerance or type 2 diabetes by the end of their fourth decade. PCOS is the single most common cause of infertility in young women and it is the underlying cause in 75% of women who have infertility due to anovulation. Source: https://cks.nice.org.uk/polycystic-ovary-syndrome#!backgroundSub:3

40 E
Pre-eclampsia occurs only in pregnancy and is of unknown aetiology although it is more common in patients with diabetes. Pre-eclampsia is defined by the new onset of elevated blood pressure and protein-uria after 20 weeks of gestation. It is considered severe if blood pressure and proteinuria are increased substantially or symptoms of end-organ damage (including foetal growth restriction) occur. The only cure is delivery, which may not be best for the baby. Labour will probably be induced if condition is mild and the woman is near term (37 to 40 weeks of pregnancy). If it is too early to deliver, the doctor will watch the health of the mother and her baby very closely. She may need medicines and bed rest at home or in the hospital to lower her blood pressure. Medicines also might be used to prevent the mother from having seizures. Source: https://www.womenshealth.gov/pregnancy/youre-pregnant-now-what/pregnancy-complications

41 D
Sertraline is safe post-MI and considered the drug of choice in these patients. However, citalopram is associated with dose-dependent QT interval prolongation and is contraindicated in patients with known QT interval prolongation or congenital long QT syndrome.

42 B

The symptoms are indicative of an ulcer. However, as the pain worsens at night this suggests duodenal ulceration. Symptoms of stomach ulcers are less consistent but often associated with weight loss. The patient is taking an NSAID which has likely precipitated the ulcer. If ulcers are suspected, referral to the GP is required as peptic ulcers can only be conclusively diagnosed via endoscopy.

43 D

Sciatica is caused by compression of one or more nerve roots in the lumbosacral spine. The compression can be caused by a herniated intervertebral disc ('slipped disc') - about 90% of cases. This most commonly occurs at the L4-L5 and L5-S1 levels. Source: https://cks.nice.org.uk/sciatica-lumbar-radiculopathy#!background Sub:2

44 B

Orlistat might affect the absorption of concurrently administered drugs - consider separating administration. Particular care should be taken with antiepileptics, antiretrovirals and drugs that have a narrow therapeutic index.

45 E

The patient is suffering from otitis media and should be managed with analgesia e.g. paracetamol or ibuprofen, unless they are systemically unwell e.g. fever.

46 A

Infectious mononucleosis or glandular fever (also known as the kissing disease because of its prevalence amongst 15–24 year olds) is sometimes misdiagnosed because of its general symptom profile. However, fatigue can linger for many months. It is caused by the *Epstein-Barr virus*. *Parovirus B19* causes erythema infectiosum (slapped cheek disease) which is most commonly found in children between the ages of 3–15 years of age. *Parainfluenza virus* causes croup and *paramyxovirus* causes mumps.

47 E

The symptoms are consistent with the classical presentation of rosacea. The first-line treatment for this condition is topical metronidazole, whereas azelaic acid is the second-line treatment. Adapelene and co-pyrindiol are used to treat acne and would not be used in cases of rosacea. Other treatments for rosacea include oral lymecycline, oxytetracycline, doxycycline, erythromycin, topical ivermectin, brimonidine or laser therapy.

48 C

One fingertip unit (FTU) is the amount of topical steroid that is squeezed out from a standard tube along an adult's fingertip before being rubbed onto a child. A fingertip is from the very end of the finger to the first crease in the finger. One FTU is used to treat an area of skin on a child equivalent to twice the size of the flat of an adult's hand with the fingers together. You can gauge the amount of topical steroid to use by using your (adult) hand to measure the amount of skin affected on the child. Two FTUs are about the same as 1 g of topical steroid. From this you can work out the amount of topical steroid to use. See guide for a 3–5 year old: https://www.pennine-gp-training.co.uk/res/Eczema%20finger%20tip%20units.pdf

49 B

Angular cheilitis can occur at any age but occurs more frequently in those wearing braces or dentures. The most common cause of angular cheilitis is a yeast infection candida. Saliva can build up and get trapped in the corners of the lips causing lips to crack. A person may lick their lips to relieve the pain or dryness of their lips, however this excess saliva accumulates in the corners creating ideal conditions for candida yeast to grow. Source: https://publicdocuments.sth.nhs.uk/pil2642.pdf

50 B

All of the other factors are known risk factors/triggers of peptic ulcers. With advanced age, the pylorus permits bile reflux into the stomach creating an environment that favours ulcer formation. Also, people with blood type O have an above normal incidence of duodenal ulcers. Gastric colonisation with *H. pylori* can cause peptic ulcers (approximately 50–70% of *H.pylori* infections cause duodenal ulcers and 30–50% cause gastric ulcers). Long term use of NSAIDs is one of the most common causes of peptic ulcers. Source: https://www.msdmanuals.com/en-gb/professional/gastrointestinal-disorders/gastritis-and-peptic-ulcer-disease/peptic-ulcer-disease

SECTION C

1 B

Grapefruit is broken down by the same cytochrome systems as statins, and therefore can lead to accumulation of metabolites and lead to increased risk of hepatic dysfunction and rhabdomyolysis.

2 D

Clarithromycin with concomitant simvastatin use leads to increased risk of rhabdomyolysis and should therefore be avoided.

3 A

Lithium is a mood-stabilising drug used most commonly prophylactically in bipolar disorder. It has a narrow therapeutic range and a long half-life. Toxicity may be precipitated by dehydration, renal failure, diuretics (especially bendroflumethiazide), ACE inhibitors, NSAIDs and metronidazole. Features of toxicity include:

- coarse tremor (a fine tremor is seen in therapeutic levels)
- hyperreflexia
- acute confusion
- seizure
- coma.

4 A

Amlodipine is not associated with increased lithium toxicity. Diuretics that promote renal sodium loss can lead to increased toxicity. ACE inhibitors reduce glomerular filtration rate and enhance tubular reabsorption of lithium thus increasing toxicity risk.

5 A

Mild-moderate toxicity may respond to volume resuscitation with normal saline. However, in severe cases, such as this with grossly elevated lithium levels and features of acutely impaired renal function, haemodialysis is required. Sodium bicarbonate is sometimes used but there is limited evidence to support this.

6 E

Allopurinol leads to a reduction of uric acid levels as it inhibits xanthine oxidase, which thus reduces uric acid production.

ANSWERS

7 D

Tell him to go to A & E for blood tests. There is a risk of agranulocytosis with carbimazole, particularly within the first 3 months of initiating treatment. It is a potentially life-threatening condition if left untreated, so he needs urgent blood tests.

8 A

Allopurinol and azathioprine should not be co-prescribed unless the combination cannot be avoided. Allopurinol interferes with the metabolism of azathioprine, increasing plasma levels of 6-mercaptopurine which may result in potentially fatal blood dyscrasias. Concomitant use requires special precautions: the dose of azathioprine should be reduced to 25% of the recommended dose and the patient's blood count should be monitored vigilantly.

9 C

NICE recommends that patients should initially be assessed in primary care using the CRB65 criteria:

- C Confusion (abbreviated mental test score <= 8/10)
- R Respiration rate >= 30/min
- B Blood pressure: systolic <= 90 mmHg and/or diastolic <= 60 mmHg
- 65 Aged >= 65 years

Patients are stratified for risk of death as follows:

- 0: low risk (less than 1% mortality risk) consider treatment at home
- 1 or 2: intermediate risk (1-10% mortality risk) consider same day assessment in hospital
- 3 or 4: high risk (more than 10% mortality risk). Require urgent admission to hospital

10 E

It is important for people with Addison's disease to increase their corticosteroid cover if they are under physical stress, such as during a period of illness to reduce the risk of adrenal crisis. It is difficult to accurately predict the needs of each person, but as a guide for adults, the person should double the normal dose of hydrocortisone (or alternative glucocorticoid) if they have a fever or are prescribed antibiotics for an infection until they are recovered.

ANSWERS

11 E

Rifampicin may cause temporary discolouration of your teeth, sweat, urine, saliva and tears (a yellow, orange, red, or brown colour). This side effect is usually not harmful.

12 C

She is out of the 72-hour window for levonorgestrel. Ulipristal acetate is licensed for use up to 120 hours post unprotected sexual intercourse, however if becomes less effective the longer it is taken after unprotected sex. The IUD is the most effective form of emergency contraception. Trials suggest the failure rate for the IUD as emergency contraception is lower than 0.1%. This means less than 1 woman in 1,000 using the IUD as emergency contraception will become pregnant. The IUD must be fitted by a healthcare professional within 5 days (120 hours) of having unprotected sex or, if it's possible to estimate when you ovulate, up to 5 days after you ovulate.

13 D

Supraventricular tachycardia (SVT) is a common heart abnormality that presents as a fast heart rate. The valsalva manoeuvre generates increased pressure within the chest cavity and aims to trigger a slowing of heart rate that may stop the abnormal rhythm. It is usually attempted first line before medications are given. See BNF, Cardiovascular system, Arrhythmias, Paroxysmal supraventricular tachycardia overview.

14 C

Cocaine is a sympathomimetic drug that causes chest pain, hypertension, agitation and arrhythmias. Hyperthermia and rhabdomyolysis are recognised complications resulting from its serotoninergic effects.

15 B

Clopidogrel irreversibly inhibits platelet aggregation via P2Y12 class ADP receptors.

16 D

SGLT2 inhibitors, also called gliflozins, are a class of medications that inhibit reabsorption of glucose in the kidney and therefore lower blood sugar. There is increased urinary excretion of glucose which can potentially increase the risk of urinary tract infections.

17 E

There are several groups of people who are eligible for the intramuscular influenza vaccine. These include people aged 65 years or over, BMI >40 and people with chronic cardiac/respiratory/liver/kidney disease. Children eligible for the flu vaccine aged between 2 and 17 will usually have the flu vaccine nasal spray. See NHS: https://www.nhs.uk/conditions/vaccinations/who-should-have-flu-vaccine/

18 B

The standard dose of a strong opioid for breakthrough pain is usually one-sixth of the regular 24-hour dose, repeated every 2–4 hours as required (up to hourly may be needed if pain is severe or in the last days of life).

19 C

Recent changes in drug regulation have meant that gabapentinoids are now classified as controlled drugs, therefore only up to 30 days' worth of medication can be given on a single prescription.

20 C

This is a medical emergency. As no IV access is already established, the fastest way to raise his blood sugar is with glucagon. Oral lucozade is not a safe option as with GCS <8 there are airway concerns.

21 A

Sulfonylureas are the most likely group of medication to cause hypoglycaemia when taken in isolation. Meglitinides are a class of drug which have a similar response as sulphonylureas but act for a shorter time. As the drugs act for a shorter period than sulphonylureas, the side effects of hypoglycaemia and weight gain have a smaller likelihood.

22 A

As per NICE guidelines, patients over the age of 55 or Afro-Caribbean's of any age should be started on a calcium channel blocker as first-line antihypertensive therapy.

23 B

An inhaled corticosteroid (ICS) should be used as preventer therapy for all people who use an inhaled SABA three times a week or more, and/or have asthma symptoms three times a week or more, and/or are woken at night by asthma symptoms once weekly or more.

24 E

Treatment of complications of tricyclic poisoning consists of correction of metabolic acidosis with sodium bicarbonate.

25 C

The combination of reduced conscious level, reduced respiratory rate and small pupils (miosis) is a classic triad for opioid misuse.

26 C

The dopamine agonists ropinirole, pramipexole and rotigotine may be used for the treatment of moderate to severe restless leg syndrome.

27 C

The patient is pregnant and with negative varicella serology, is at risk of varicella infection with risks to the unborn baby also. Varicella zoster immunoglobulin transfers passive immunity and reduces the risk of acquiring infection. If she develops chickenpox there is a high risk of adverse outcome, therefore management cannot wait until she develops chickenpox.

28 D

The combination of nitrates (and drugs such as nicorandil) with sildenafil is contraindicated. This combination must be avoided as it can produce significant hypotension and is potentially fatal.

29 B

The history suggests this patient may be dehydrated. Morphine is renally excreted, thus acute renal failure can lead to toxicity.

30 C

Naloxone should be given to patients to reverse the effects of opioid toxicity. Flumazenil is a drug given to reverse cases of benzodiazepine overdose.

31 D

This is an absolute contraindication to starting the combined pill due to increased risk of stroke. Please refer to the UKMEC summary for a detailed breakdown of full guidance around different medical conditions and their impact on the prescription of contraceptives.

32 B

Irregular periods often occur when taking the progestogen-only pill compared with the combined oral contraceptive which is useful in the management of dysmenorrhoea.

33 A

Older brands of the progestogen-only pill have a 3-hour window. Newer brands such as *Cerelle*® and *Cerazette*® contain desogestrel giving them a 12-hour window. Please also note that *Femulen*® and *Micronor*® have been discontinued in the NHS.

34 D

35 E

When paracetamol is metabolised it produces a toxic metabolite. This is normally bound by glutathione which becomes saturated in overdose. N-acetylcysteine acts to replenish this.

36 E

N-acetylcysteine IV is still the treatment of choice and can be effective up to, and possibly beyond, 24 hours of overdose.

37 D

This is in keeping with NICE guidelines. When topical treatment has failed, options include an oral antifungal treatment. Terbinafine is generally better tolerated and has fewer interactions than griseofulvin and itraconazole, but it is not suitable for all people (such as children and people with chronic or active liver disease).

38 E

Using an SSRI together with naproxen may increase the risk of bleeding. The interaction may be more likely if the patient is elderly or has kidney or liver disease.

ANSWERS

39 C
SSRIs alone increase the risk of gastrointestinal adverse effects. They block the reuptake of serotonin by the thrombocytes, resulting in an impairment of the haemostatic function. This when used with NSAIDs increases the risk of bleeding.

40 C

41 E
Varenicline (brand name *Champix*®) is a medicine that works in two ways. It reduces cravings for nicotine like NRT, but it also blocks the rewarding and reinforcing effects of smoking. Evidence suggests it is the most effective medication to help people stop smoking. However, it should be used in caution in those with a history of psychiatric illness as it may exacerbate underlying mental health condition. It has also been shown that it may predispose to seizures or lower seizure threshold.

42 E
Supportive therapy is the mainstay of treatment in *Cryptosporidium* diarrhoea.

43 C
Tetracyclines are associated with photosensitivity reactions.

44 B
Acne vulgaris is a common skin disorder which usually occurs in adolescence. A simple step-up management scheme often used in the treatment of acne is as follows:

- Single topical therapy (topical retinoids, benzoyl peroxide)
- Topical combination therapy (topical antibiotic, benzoyl peroxide, topical retinoid)
- Oral antibiotics e.g. oxytetracycline, doxycycline. Improvement may not be seen for 3-4 months.
- Oral isotretinoin: only under specialist guidance

45 B
The exact mechanism of action of isotretinoin is unknown. However, it has been found to decrease the size and activity of sebaceous glands,

which decreases secretion and probably explains the rapid clinical improvement. As a consequence, many people suffer from dry skin and lips.

46 D

Isotretinoin is a known teratogen, and hence all women considered to be at risk of conceiving will be entered into the Pregnancy Prevention Programme whilst taking their course of isotretinoin, in order to minimise the risk of pregnancy. Each month women are asked to attend the clinic for a pregnancy test and will have a final pregnancy test 5 weeks after finishing treatment. Women will only be supplied with 30 days of treatment on each visit following a negative pregnancy test and prescriptions for isotretinoin must be collected from the pharmacy within 7 days of it being signed by the doctor.

47 D

The BNF states 'breast-feeding is acceptable with all antiepileptic drugs, taken in normal doses, with the possible exception of barbiturates'.

48 B

Cradle cap or seborrhoeic dermatitis is a relatively common skin disorder seen in children. It is characterised by an erythematous rash with coarse yellow scales. Management depends on severity:

- Mild-moderate: baby shampoo and baby oils
- Severe: mild topical steroids e.g. 1% hydrocortisone

49 D

Scabies is an intensely itchy skin infestation caused by the human parasite *Sarcoptes scabiei*. Permethrin 5% cream is first-line treatment, then malathion aqueous 0.5% if permethrin is contraindicated or not tolerated.

50 C

The product should usually be applied to the whole body from the chin and ears downwards, paying special attention to the areas between the fingers and toes and under the nails. Permethrin should be washed off after 8 to 12 hours, and malathion after 24 hours. A second application is required one week after the first.

51 C

Promoting pharmacy in the media and government is not a role of the GPhC. This is for the Royal Pharmaceutical Society.

52 E

Pharmacy professionals should recognise their own values, but never impose them on other people.

53 D

For people who have mild-to-moderate C. *difficile* infection, consult local policy or discuss further management with a microbiologist and consider prescribing an antibiotic. As a guide, Public Health England recommends:

- For the initial episode of mild-to-moderate C. *difficile* infection: oral metronidazole 400 mg three times a day for 10–14 days.
- Vancomycin and fidaxomicin are reserved for severe C. *difficile* infection or for subsequent recurrences.

Source: https://cks.nice.org.uk/diarrhoea-antibiotic-associated #!scenario

54 E

Simple calculation of $65 \times 20\,\text{mg/kg} = 1300\,\text{mg}$.

55 D

According to SPC, sodium chloride 0.9% injection or glucose 5% are suitable.

56 C

'Red man syndrome' is commonly known with fast vancomycin infusion.

57 C

The diagnosis here is neuroleptic malignant syndrome which can be precipitated by either high doses of a single anti-psychotic medication, but more commonly by the use of combinations of anti-psychotic medication.

58 B

As this is the first occasion that this is found, the correct thing to do is offer lifestyle advice and repeat the measurement.

59 E

Use simple pain ladder which states paracetamol as step 1. Source: https://cks.nice.org.uk/analgesia-mild-to-moderate-pain#!scenario

60 A

A pain at the back of the ankle is most likely an Achilles heel pain. This is the only option that is reasonable to deduce from the options.

61 D

Refer to GP as Achilles tendon rupture requires further treatment, possibly with a brace to help aid recovery.

62 E

This sample shows hyperkalaemia, mild hyponatraemia, a normal chloride and bicarbonate concentration with a raised urea and normal creatinine. The only explanation for this is the diuretic therapy. Spironolactone is known to induce hyperkalaemia, and when mixed with other antidiuretics can also present hyponatremia.

63 B

He has impaired glucose tolerance and should be given advice as he is at risk of developing diabetes.

64 D

Norovirus affects adults and children. Rotavirus is usually only present in children. The other viruses are either mild in single symptoms, or not relevant. See NHS: https://www.nhs.uk/conditions/norovirus/

65 C

A peak flow test is the most useful initial measurement to know whether it is the airways that have constricted, then appropriate asthmatic management can be given. See NHS: https://www.nhs.uk/conditions/peak-flow-test/

66 D

The negative predictive value is the probability that a subject who tests negative for a condition actually does not have the condition. There were 95 people who were tested negative and did not have the condition. However, there were 5 patients who tested negative who actually did have the condition. Therefore, the test is correct 95 out of 100 times, which is then calculated as the negative predictive value of 95%.

67 D
Metformin is contraindicated in significant renal impairment as it can cause lactic acidosis. It does not cause hypoglycaemia (unlike gliclazide, a sulphonylurea) and is an ideal first choice in obese patients. This patient is obese and therefore gliclazide is unsuitable for this patient as it causes weight gain. Rosiglitazone is used as an adjunct to biguanides or sulphonylureas, never alone and never with insulin. Insulin glargine is not appropriate as a first-line medication. If the option of diet control and exercise was offered, it would be a reasonable first line in many patients. This patient's fasting glucose is significantly raised (9 mmols) and this patient is likely to need pharmacological management.

68 B
Adrenaline 150 mcg is for children weighing up to 25 kg. *EpiPen Junior*® is available in the NHS (0.3 mL/0.15 mg adrenaline).

69 C
Refer to vinblastine SPC for wording on routes of administration.

70 D
Soft blue cheese should be avoided as according to NHS website. Source: https://www.nhs.uk/conditions/pregnancy-and-baby/foods-to-avoid-pregnant/

Extended matching
answers

SECTION A

1 F
   Common or very common side effect of gliclazide.

2 A
   See BNF, Blood and nutrition, Calcium imbalance overview.

3 H
   See BNF, Nervous system, Antidepressant drugs overview.

4 C
   See BNF monograph for enalapril maleate.

5 G
   See BNF monograph for furosemide.

6 E
   See NHS: https://www.nhs.uk/conditions/psoriasis/

7 H
   See NHS: https://www.nhs.uk/conditions/athletes-foot/

8 F
   See NHS: https://www.nhs.uk/conditions/shingles/

9 A
   See CKS: https://cks.nice.org.uk/acne-vulgaris#!diagnosisSub

ANSWERS

10 C
See NHS: https://www.nhs.uk/conditions/atopic-eczema/

11 D
See NHS: https://www.nhs.uk/conditions/glaucoma/

12 F
See NHS: https://www.nhs.uk/conditions/red-eye/

13 G
See NHS: https://www.nhs.uk/conditions/uveitis/

14 A
See NHS: https://www.nhs.uk/conditions/conjunctivitis/

15 B
See NHS: https://www.nhs.uk/conditions/conjunctivitis/

16 D
See BNF, Endocrine system, Diabetes, pregnancy and breast-feeding overview.

17 F
Patient is overweight, therefore metformin is appropriate. See SPC: https://www.medicines.org.uk/emc/product/594/smpc

18 B
Sulphonylureas associated with moderate weight gain. See BNF, Endocrine system, Type 2 diabetes overview.

19 G
See BNF monograph for pioglitazone.

20 A
See BNF monograph for empagliflozin.

21 B
See BNF monograph for aspirin.

22 C
See BNF monograph for clopidogrel.

23 H

See BNF monograph for warfarin.

24 D

See BNF monograph for dalteparin sodium.

25 H

DOACs increase risk of thromboembolic events for patients with history of this syndrome - see BNF monograph for apixaban for explanation.

26 C

See BNF, Infection, Lyme disease overview.

27 H

28 G

See BNF monograph for metronidazole and CKS: https://cks.nice .org.uk/bacterial-vaginosis#!scenario

29 D

See CKS: https://cks.nice.org.uk/cellulitis-acute#!scenario
Recommendation:2

30 A

See CKS: https://cks.nice.org.uk/chest-infections-adult#!scenario
Recommendation:3

31 E

See BNF monograph for flucloxacillin.

32 H

Avoid all forms of tetracyclines in under 12 years olds due to contraindication. See BNF monograph for tetracycline.

33 F

See BNF monograph for gentamicin.

34 C

35 B

Tendon damage risk with use of quinolones. See BNF monograph for ciprofloxacin.

36 H

37 E

38 D
See BNF monograph for lofepramine.

39 G
See BNF, Nervous system, Antidepressant drugs overview.

40 C
See BNF monograph for lithium carbonate.

41 E
See BNF, Appendix 1: Interactions, Verapamil.

42 A
See BNF, Cardiovascular system, Hypertension overview.

43 F
See BNF, Cardiovascular system, Hypertension overview.

44 G
See BNF, Cardiovascular system, Hypertension overview.

45 B
See BNF monograph for bisoprolol fumarate.

46 D

47 A

48 G

49 C

50 H
See FSRH: https://www.fsrh.org/standards-and-guidance/documents/ukmec-2016/

SECTION B

1 D

Giardia is a leading but treatable cause of infectious gastroenteritis worldwide. Most patients with *Giardia* in the UK acquire their infection in the UK and not from overseas travel. Symptoms are consistent with gastroenteritis. Source: https://www.bmj.com/content/bmj/355/bmj.i5369.full.pdf

2 E

The head louse is an obligate ectoparasite that causes head lice infestations. Head lice is very common in children and slightly more common in girls due to longer hair. Lice do not jump, they crawl from one head to another which is why children playing in close proximity often catch lice. The empty egg shells (nits) of lice may be confused with dandruff as it is white in appearance.

3 E

The severity of infestation varies from a few lice (less than 10) to over 100 lice (in up to 5% of people) and more than 1000 in severe cases, but a typical infestation might have about 30 lice per head. Source: https://cks.nice.org.uk/head-lice#!backgroundSub

4 H

Trichomoniasis is a sexually transmitted infection (STI) caused by the flagellated protozoan *Trichomonas vaginalis*. Transmission of *Trichomonas vaginalis* is almost exclusively through sexual intercourse. Vertical transmission can occur from an infected mother to baby during vaginal delivery. Source: https://cks.nice.org.uk/trichomoniasis#!background

5 F

Scabies is an intensely itchy skin infestation caused by the human parasite *Sarcoptes scabiei*, a 0.3 to 0.5 mm mite that burrows into the epidermis and tunnels through the stratum corneum. Source: https://cks.nice.org.uk/scabies#!backgroundSub

6 F

The first-line treatment for non-crusted scabies is the topical insecticide permethrin 5% cream, and crotamiton 10% may be prescribed to soothe pruritus which may last several weeks after infection has been cleared.

ANSWERS

7 C

Enterobius vermicularis (threadworm) is the most common worm infection. Night time perianal itching is the classic presentation. The associated itch is caused by the mucus produced by females when laying eggs and causes an allergic type reaction to the skin. Other symptoms include local tickling sensation or acute pain, and any child with high time perianal itching is very likely to have threadworm.

8 G

A toxoplasma infection can occur via several routes including through cats:

- Accidentally swallowing the parasite through contact with cat faeces that contain toxoplasma
- Toxoplasma which could happen by cleaning a cat's litter box when the cat has shed toxoplasma in its faeces and not washing hands sufficiently afterwards
- Touching or ingesting anything that has come into contact with cat faeces that contains toxoplasma
- Accidentally ingesting contaminated soil e.g., not washing hands after gardening or eating unwashed fruits or vegetables from a garden

9 G

Varicella vaccine is used to prevent chickenpox; however it is not available via the NHS due to concerns that it could increase the risk of chickenpox and shingles in adults. However, it is offered to individuals who are likely to come into contact with people particularly vulnerable to chickenpox, such as those having chemotherapy. This reduces the risk of chickenpox spreading to vulnerable people.

10 A

Currently, the national NHS HPV vaccination programme uses a vaccine called *Gardasil*®. *Gardasil*® protects against four types of HPV: 6, 11, 16 and 18. Between them, types 16 and 18 are the cause of most cervical cancers in the UK (more than 70%). HPV types 6 and 11 cause around 90% of genital warts, therefore *Gardasil*® helps protect girls against both cervical cancer and genital warts.

11 E

Patients who have had their spleen removed are more susceptible to pneumococcal infections.

12 D

It is recommended that pregnant women receive the pertussis vaccine to help protect their babies from whooping cough from 16 weeks up to 32 weeks pregnant.

13 F

The oral rotavirus vaccine is given as two doses for babies aged 8 and 12 weeks alongside their other routine childhood vaccinations to protect against the rotavirus infection, which is a common cause of gastroenteritis, diarrhoea and sickness in infants.

14 F

Ondansetron is from a group of 5-HT$_3$ receptor antagonists (others include: granisetron, tropisetron, dolasetron, and palonosetron) used to relieve symptoms of chemotherapy-induced nausea.

15 E

Dexamethasone acts synergistically with 5HT$_3$-receptor antagonists to potentiate the anti-emetic effect.

16 A

5-fluorouracil may produce palmar-plantar erythrodysaesthesia (hand-foot syndrome) that results in a dry, reddened and painful area on the extremities of the hands and feet.

17 H

Trastuzumab is indicated for early breast cancer and metastatic stages as monotherapy, or in combination depending on prior treatment of patient etc. Trastuzumab should only be used in patients with tumours that have HER2 overexpression or HER2 gene amplification.

18 G

In breast cancer patients, at the tumour level, tamoxifen acts primarily as an antioestrogen, preventing oestrogen binding to the oestrogen receptor. Tamoxifen reduces but does not eliminate the risk of breast cancer. In clinical trials, tamoxifen decreased the incidence of oestrogen receptor-positive tumours but did not alter the incidence of oestrogen receptor-negative tumours. The use of tamoxifen should be as part of a program including regular breast surveillance tailored to the individual woman, taking into account her risk of breast cancer. Tamoxifen is indicated for:

- the treatment of breast cancer
- the treatment of anovulatory infertility.

19 G

In selected patients, the use of tamoxifen with prophylactic anticoagulation may be justified as there is a two- to three-fold increase in the risk for VTE in healthy tamoxifen-treated women. Thus, in patients with breast cancer, prescribers should obtain careful histories with respect to the patient's personal and family history of VTE.

20 D

Cisplatin causes ototoxicity in 31% of patients treated with a single dose of 50 mg/m^2 and is manifested by tinnitus and/or hearing loss. It is unclear whether cisplatin induced ototoxicity is reversible, thus careful monitoring by audiometry should be performed prior to initiation of therapy and prior to subsequent doses of cisplatin.

21 A

Gastrointestinal side effects are very common with 5-flourouracil and treatment should only be continued once the patient has fully recovered from stomatitis, diarrhoea, bleeding, vomiting etc.

22 B

Anastrozole is indicated for the treatment of hormone receptor-positive advanced breast cancer in postmenopausal women. Anastrozole should not be used in premenopausal women.

23 G

These symptoms are consistent with rosacea, and metronidazole should be prescribed as first-line treatment for this condition. Rosacea is sometimes confused for acne, however, occurs more frequently in middle-aged adults. Also, the bulbous nose (rhinophyma) and red cheeks are characteristic of severe rosacea.

24 B

Benzoyl peroxide is an established and effective keratolytic agent with antibacterial properties. It has been shown to be effective in reducing the local population of *Propionibacterium acnes* leading to a reduction in the production of irritant fatty acids in the sebaceous glands. Source: https://www.medicines.org.uk/emc/product/2225/smpc#PHARMACOLOGICAL_PROPS

25 C

Co-cyprindiol (*Dianette*®) or other ethinylestradiol/cyproterone acetate containing products may be considered in moderate to severe acne where other treatments have failed but require careful discussion of the risks and benefits with the patient. Use should be discontinued 3 months after acne has been controlled and prescription guided by the UK Medical Eligibility Criteria for Contraceptive Use and the Summary of Product Characteristics for the individual product. Source: https://cks.nice.org.uk/acne-vulgaris#!scenarioRecommendation

26 A

Amorolfine 5% w/v medicated nail lacquer should be applied to the affected finger or toenails once weekly. Before the first application, it is essential that the affected areas of nail (particularly the nail surfaces) should be filed down as thoroughly as possible using a nail file. The surface of the nail should then be cleansed and degreased using a cleaning swab and treatment duration usually lasts for 6 months for fingernails and 9 to 12 months for toenails. Source: https://www.medicines.org.uk/emc/product/8053/pil

27 H

Selenium sulphide (*Selsun*® shampoo 2.5%) is used to manage simple dandruff and seborrhoeic dermatitis of the scalp. Selenium sulphide appears to have a cytostatic effect on cells of the epidermis and follicular epithelium, thus reducing corneocyte production. *Selsun*® acts as an antiseborrhoeic agent which effectively controls itching and scaling dandruff.

28 F

Ketoconazole 2% w/w shampoo is indicated for the treatment and prevention of seborrhoeic dermatitis, pityriasis capitis (dandruff) and pityriasis versicolor that may be associated with the fungus

Pityrosporum. Ketoconazole is a synthetic imidazole-dioxalane derivative. It is a broad-spectrum antifungal agent which inhibits the growth of common dermatophytes and yeasts by altering the permeability of the cell membrane. Source: https://www.medicines.org.uk/emc/product/4559/smpc#PHARMACODYNAMIC_PROPS

29 E

For women of childbearing potential, the prescription duration of isotretinoin capsules should ideally be limited to 30 days in order to support regular follow-up, including pregnancy testing and monitoring. Ideally, pregnancy testing, issuing a prescription and dispensing of isotretinoin capsules should occur on the same day. Dispensing of isotretinoin should occur within a maximum of 7 days of the prescription. This monthly follow-up will allow ensuring that regular pregnancy testing and monitoring is performed and that the patient is not pregnant before receiving the next cycle of medication. Source: https://www.medicines.org.uk/emc/product/3870/smpc#CLINICAL_PRECAUTIONS

30 E

Isotretinoin has been associated with an increase in plasma triglyceride levels. Isotretinoin should be discontinued if hypertriglyceridaemia cannot be controlled at an acceptable level or if symptoms of pancreatitis occur. Elevated serum lipid values usually return to normal on reduction of the dose or discontinuation of treatment and may also respond to dietary measures. Levels in excess of 800 mg/dL or 9 mmol/L are sometimes associated with acute pancreatitis, which may be fatal. Source: https://www.medicines.org.uk/emc/product/3870/smpc#CLINICAL_PRECAUTIONS

31 D

Hydrocortisone preparations are usually well tolerated, but if any signs of hypersensitivity appear, application should stop immediately. Striae may occur especially in intertriginous areas. Source: https://www.medicines.org.uk/emc/product/4600/smpc#UNDESIRABLE_EFFECTS

32 E

Digoxin maintenance dosage should be based upon the percentage of the peak body stores lost each day through elimination.

The following formula has had wide clinical use: Maintenance dose = peak body stores × (% daily loss / 100). When switching from intravenous to oral route, may need to increase dose by 20–33% to maintain the same plasma-digoxin concentration.

33 H

Simvastatin, like other inhibitors of HMG-CoA reductase, occasionally causes myopathy manifested as muscle pain, tenderness or weakness with creatine kinase (CK) above ten times the upper limit of normal (ULN). All patients starting therapy with simvastatin, or whose dose of simvastatin is being increased, should be advised of the risk of myopathy and told to report promptly any unexplained muscle pain, tenderness or weakness. Caution should be exercised in patients with pre-disposing factors for rhabdomyolysis. In order to establish a reference baseline value, a CK level should be measured before starting a treatment in the following situations:

- Elderly (age ≥ 65 years)
  - Female gender
- Renal impairment
- Uncontrolled hypothyroidism
- Personal or familial history of hereditary muscular disorders
- Previous history of muscular toxicity with a statin or fibrate
- Alcohol abuse

Source: https://www.medicines.org.uk/emc/product/7166/smpc

34 F

Loop diuretics such as furosemide is recommended for use in all indications where a prompt and effective diuresis is required. Furosemide improves some haemodynamic parameters and dyspnoea due to congestion e.g. water and salt retention. Source: https://www.medicines.org.uk/emc/product/5867/smpc

35 C

Cangrelor is a direct P2Y12 platelet receptor antagonist that blocks adenosine diphosphate-induced platelet activation and aggregation. It is intended for specialised use in an acute and hospital setting (under expert supervision) and is given in combination with aspirin for the reduction of thrombotic cardiovascular events in patients with coronary artery disease undergoing percutaneous coronary intervention (PCI) who have not received an oral P2Y12 inhibitor (e.g. clopidogrel, prasugrel, ticagrelor) prior to the PCI procedure, and in whom oral therapy with a P2Y12 inhibitor is not suitable.

36 E
Digoxin is indicated for the treatment of congestive heart failure and may be used for certain supraventricular dysrhythmias, particularly atrial fibrillation. It is a cardiac glycoside that increases the force of myocardial contraction and reduces conductivity within the atrioventricular (AV) node.

37 A
Amiodarone is used to treat arrhythmias, particularly when other drugs are ineffective or contra-indicated. It can cause both hypo- and hyperthyroidism. In this instance the patient is showing signs of hypothyroidism and concomitant levothyroxine should be considered.

38 G
A cough that persists for more than 3 weeks and is accompanied by night sweats is indicative of TB which is caused by the pathogen *Mycobacterium tuberculosis*. It qualifies as a notifiable disease and must be reported to the local health protection teams as it is a highly contagious and serious disease. Source: http://www .blackpooljsna.org.uk/Living-and-Working-Well/Health-Protection/ Infectious-and-communicable-diseases.aspx

39 E
Methicillin-resistant Staphylococcus aureus (MRSA) are strains of *S. aureus* which have developed resistance to a number of commonly used antibiotics including ß-lactam antibiotics. It is usually acquired following direct or indirect contact with healthcare services and is more likely to occur in older age groups. Admission to hospital or other contact with healthcare services such as for acute or chronic disease management (including use of invasive devices, for example, urinary catheters) increases risk. Definition of MRSA based on where infection is likely to have been acquired (hospital vs community) is becoming less relevant as crossover in strain types identified in

hospital and the community becomes increasingly common. Source: https://cks.nice.org.uk/mrsa-in-primary-care#!backgroundSub:1

40 F
Moraxella catarrhalis is one of the most common bacterial causes of otitis media in children. Source: https://www.msdmanuals.com/en-gb/professional/infectious-diseases/gram-negative-cocci-and-coccobacilli/moraxella-catarrhalis-infection

41 A
Bordetella pertussis causes whooping cough that is characterised by cough fits (paroxysm) which consists of short expiratory burst followed by an inspiratory gasp making the characteristic whooping sound. It is more common in children but can occur in adults. May be severe enough to cause cyanosis in children and is frequently associated with post-tussive vomiting. Adults may experience sweating attacks with facial flushing, and, rarely, cough syncope. Source: https://cks.nice.org.uk/whooping-cough#!diagnosisSub

42 H
Respiratory syncytial virus (RSV) infection in children is one of the major viral causes of childhood acute lower respiratory disease. It is so common that most children have been infected with the virus by age 2. Complications are rare but can lead to bronchiolitis.

43 B
The *Epstein-Barr virus* is responsible for glandular fever as described in the question and easily spreads through human contact, especially via the saliva.

44 C
The symptoms are characteristic of cystitis which is most commonly caused by *Escherichia coli*. The bacteria ascend through the urethra and into the bladder.

45 H
The child is suffering from Reye's syndrome. In this case the mother used aspirin to treat the high fever mentioned, however this aspirin use is not explicitly stated. A clue lies in the discussion between the pharmacist and patient's mother over recent medication history.

Reye's syndrome is rare but most often occurs when the child is recovering from a viral infection, most commonly the flu or chickenpox. Source: https://patient.info/doctor/reyes-syndrome-pro

46 E

The infant has meningitis as indicated by the nature and swift onset of symptoms. Meningitis is caused by a viral or bacterial infection, although viral is much more common. The infection causes inflammation in the meninges that protect the brain and spinal cord and can be fatal if not treated promptly. Meningitis is uncommon due to the Hib vaccine but when it does occur peak incidence is between 6–12 months. Signs and symptoms are non-specific and flu-like in the early stages but in the later stages of the disease a petechial or purpuric rash is characteristic along with bulging fontanel (the soft spot on top of the head) which may be due to increased pressure or fluid in the brain. Other symptoms which may appear include:

- a stiff body with jerky movements or else floppy and lifeless
- unusual grunting sounds
- vomiting/refusing to feed
- irritable when picking up, with a high pitched or moaning cry
- blotchy skin, getting paler or turning blue
- pain/irritability from muscle aches or severe limb/joint pain
- cold hands and feet
- high temperature (warning - could be normal or low in babies under 3 months)
- very sleepy/staing/expression/too sleepy to wake up
- breathing fast/difficulty breathing
- extreme shivering
- 'pin prick' rash/marks or purple bruises anywhere on the body
- sometimes diarrhoea

Source: https://www.meningitis.org/meningitis/check-symptoms/babies

47 C

For mild impetigo NICE recommends treat with topical fusidic acid (three times a day for 5 days). Topical mupirocin should only be used if impetigo is known to be caused by MRSA. If impetigo is more widespread or bullous, treat with an oral antibiotic.

48 F

Molluscum contagiosum is a common and generally harmless condition that causes spots on skin. It is most common in children and young adults and is caused by a pox virus, thus can spread to others if the spots are in direct contact with someone else. Confirmation of molluscum contagiosum does not usually require diagnostic investigations because of its classical appearance - the central umbilication (dimple). Source: https://cks.nice.org.uk/molluscum-contagiosum#!diagnosisSub

49 B

Glandular fever (infectious mononucleosis) is caused by the *Epstein-Barr virus* and is most common in young people between the ages of 15–24. It is transmitted from close salivary contact which is why it is colloquially referred to as the kissing disease. Sore throat appears in up to 90% of patients and is usually severe. It is sometimes misdiagnosed as strep-throat, thus if a sore throat persists after treatment with antibiotics it is highly suggestive of glandular fever. Source: https://cks.nice.org.uk/glandular-fever-infectious-mononucleosis#!diagnosisSub

50 D

The child has Koplik's spots which is indicative of measles. These distinct eruptions consist of small, irregular spots, and in the centre of each bright red spot there is a minute bluish white speck. These red spots with accompanying specks of a bluish colour are absolutely pathognomonic of beginning measles, and when seen it is likely that the skin rash will soon appear. Source: https://www.ncbi.nlm.nih.gov/pmc/articles/PMC2645467/

ANSWERS

SECTION C

1 C

An equal risk ratio will be 1 if the outcomes are the same in each group.

2 D

From the confidence intervals in the image, 2.05 and 5.13, 5.13 is the higher one.

3 E

Refer to the risk ratio in the Nauck study.

4 A

Refer to the test for overall effect: $Z = 5.02$ ($p < 0.00001$).

5 H

Total events 400 (metformin + sulphonylurea) + 169 (Metformin + GLP-1) = 569.

6 D

Low-molecular-weight heparins are indicated for quick anticoagulation with suspected DVT.

7 J

Warfarin is still standard of care for medium- to long-term management of these patients.

8 B

There is a significant interaction according to the BNF.

9 I

Vitamin K is the antidote for warfarin treatment as warfarin is a vitamin K antagonist.

10 G

Section 4.2 of the SPC states that 'Control is established with INR monitoring at regular intervals and subsequent warfarin maintenance dosage further adjusted according to the results obtained.' See SPC: https://www.medicines.org.uk/emc/product/3064/smpc

11 B

Cetirizine is convenient for the patient because of daily dosing and does not cause drowsiness.

12 G

13 A

This is the next line of therapy to reduce inflammation of the airways.

14 F

Information on steroid nasal sprays are available on the NHS website. See NHS: https://www.nhs.uk/conditions/steroid-nasal-sprays/

15 H

This is a common decongestant that is used to clear the airways from mucus.

16 I

Refer to the following resource for guidance on healthcare statistics: https://www.cebm.net/2014/03/number-needed-to-treat-nnt/

17 D

See definitions and examples: https://www.statisticshowto.data sciencecentral.com/probability-and-statistics/statistics-definitions/

18 J

19 A

20 B

21 H

NHS prescription validity can be found in the MEP, or online at https://www.nhs.uk/common-health-questions/medicines/how-long-is-a-prescription-valid-for/

22 F

See MEP summary table on controlled drugs.

23 D
Dosing for methotrexate is in line with NICE guidelines for rheumatoid arthritis: https://cks.nice.org.uk/dmards#!scenario:10

24 A
Refer to NICE CG62 Antenatal care for uncomplicated pregnancy, Section 1.3.2.1.

25 C
Phenobarbital has recently been reclassified and therefore has the same rules as schedule 4 and 5 controlled drugs.

26 F
Refer to any endocrinology textbook for these definitions.

27 G

28 I

29 J

30 E

Calculation answers

SECTION A

1 1 bottle

Taking 5 mL QDS, thus 20 mL per day, therefore 100 mL over the course of the week. Only needs 1 bottle to be supplied

2 75 mg

A number to the power of 0.5 is the same as the square root of that number i.e. BSA = ([height (cm) × weight (kg)] ÷ 3600)$^{0.5}$= $\sqrt{}$([height (cm) × weight (kg)] ÷ 3600) therefore, BSA = $\sqrt{}$(148 × 72] ÷ 3600) = $\sqrt{}$2.96 = 1.7205

Dose = 45 mg/m^2 × 1.7505 m^2 = 77.4225 mg

Rounded to nearest 5 mg = 75 mg

3 534 tablets

Generally easier to draw up a table to calculate the dose

Dose	No. tabs per day	No. days	Total no. tabs
60 mg	12	6	72
55 mg	11	7	77
50 mg	10	7	70
45 mg	9	7	63
40 mg	8	7	56
35 mg	7	7	49

(continued)

(*continued*)

Dose	No. tabs per day	No. days	Total no. tabs
30 mg	6	7	42
25 mg	5	7	35
20 mg	4	7	28
15 mg	3	7	21
10 mg	2	7	14
5 mg	1	7	7
		Total	534

4   875 mg
Dose = 15 mg/kg × 56 kg = 840 mg
Tablets are available in 250 mg strength, which are scored and can be halved (125 mcg)
To find number of tablets: 840 mg ÷ 125 mg/half = 6.72 halves
Therefore, round up to 7 halves
Dose to prescribe = 125 mg × 7 = 875 mg
Check it is not an overdose (max 20 mg/kg) by working out mg/kg: 875 mg ÷ 56 kg = 15.625 mg

5   46 mL
The BNF states that 92 mg in oral suspension is equivalent to 100 mg in capsules
Thus, 276 mg (92 × 3) of solution is needed per 300 mg dose
There is only one strength of oral suspension in the BNF: 30 mg/5 mL
30 mg/5 mL = 6 mg/mL
Therefore, 276 mg ÷ 6 mg/mL = 46 mL

6   250 mg
BNF states that 125 mg suppositories equivalent to 100 mg oral
Supporting information for suppositories also states to give these four times a day, not twice
Therefore, first thing to do is work out current total daily dose: 400 mg × 2 = 800 mg
Work out equivalent daily dose: 800 mg × 1.25 = 1000 mg
Thus, if given QDS, the individual dose is: 1000 ÷ 4 = 250 mg

7 81 capsules
   1 capsule on day 1
   2 capsules on day 2
   Then 3 capsules each day for another 26 days (28 − 2) = 78 capsules
   Total = 78 + 2 + 1 = 81 capsules

8 255 ampoules
   Will need to use 1 ampoule to make up each dose of ceftazidime
   Will also use 2 ampoules per dose for the flushes
   Therefore, 3 ampoules of 0.9% sodium chloride per dose = 6 ampoules per day
   Thus, 6 × (6 × 7) = 252 ampoules
   Round up to 255

9 312 tablets
   Need 2 tablets per dose (2 × 480 = 960)
   Equivalent to 4 tablets per dosing day (2 × BD)
   Only taken three times a week, so will have 4 × 3 = 12 tablets per week
   Thus, need to supply 12 × 26 = 312 tablets for the period

10 4 packs
    He will take 3 tablets on five days of the week
    He will take 4 tablets on two days of the week
    Therefore, (3 × 5) + (4 × 2) = 23 tablets per week
    Thus, 23 × 4 = 92 tablets in total
    92 ÷ 28 = 3.2857 packs

11 3 minutes
    The 100 mg/10 mL vancomycin solution is equivalent to 10 mg/mL
    Therefore, there is 30 mg of vancomycin in the patient's line when locked
    Section 4.2 of the SPC states the maximum rate of infusion is 10 mg/minute
    Therefore, the shortest time over which to flush the line lock would be 3 minutes

12 1920 mg
    From the SPC, each 16 mg of trimethoprim is accompanied with 80 mg sulfamethoxazole

If 80 ÷ 16 = 5 mg of sulfamethoxazole for every 1 mg of trimethoprim
There will be 75 mg of sulfamethoxazole for every 15 mg of trimethoprim (5 × 15 = 75)
The total dose will be 90 mg/kg/day in three divided doses (15 mg + 75 mg = 90 mg)
Thus, each individual dose will be 30 mg/kg
30 mg/kg × 63.4 kg = 1902 mg per dose
Check if needs to be rounded: 1902 mg ÷ 96 mg/mL = 19.8125 mL
Therefore, should use 20 mL per dose: 20 mL × 96 mg/mL = 1920 mg per dose
If calculated the total daily dose, then divided by 3 the same answer is obtained:
90 mg/kg/day × 63.4 kg = 5706 mg/day
5706 mg/day ÷ 3/day = 1902 mg per dose that rounds to 1920 mg

13 417 mg/kg
Each tablet of co-codamol contains 500 mg paracetamol – candidates would be expected to know this
Therefore, 60 tablets × 500 mg/tablet = 30,000 mg
He weighs 72 kg, therefore: 30,000 mg ÷ 72 kg = 416.6667 mg/kg
Round up to 417

14 Answer = 360 mg
Work out ideal body weight first: 45.5 kg + (2.3 × 3) = 52.4 kg
Dose = 52.4 kg × 7 mg/kg = 366.8 mg
Round to 40 mg: 366.8 mg ÷ 40 mg = 9.17
Therefore, to nearest 40 mg = 9 × 40 = 360 mg

15 49 tablets
3 tablets per day for 7 days = 21 tablets
2 tablets per day for 7 days = 14 tablets
Then 1 tablet per day for 14 more days = 14 tablets
Thus, 21 + 14 + 14 = 49 tablets

16 31.05 mg/mL
Absorbance is on the Y axis, and concentration on the X axis
Therefore, the equation is: $0.701 = 0.02 X + 0.08$
Rearrange to find X: $X = (0.701 - 0.08) ÷ 0.02$
Concentration is therefore 31.05 mg/mL

17 34 minutes

For mean, you add all the values together, then divide by the number of values

$(35 + 45 + 22 + 34 + 28 + 54 + 12 + 33 + 36 + 41) \div 10$

$= 340 \div 10 = 34$ minutes

18 63 cans

In order to make a sufficient supply, need to assume he is using up to 3 cans per day

Therefore, 3 cans $\times$ 21 days = 63 cans

19 1120 mg

Section 5.2 of the SPC discusses the pharmacokinetics of the drug

For teicoplanin, this section clearly states that it obeys linear pharmacokinetics

Linear pharmacokinetics is the same as first order kinetics

Therefore, if you increase the dose by X%, the serum concentration should also increase proportionally by X%

Work out percentage difference between drug level

$([20 - 16.3] \div 16.3) \times 100 = 22.6994\%$

Increase this dose by 22.6994% (will need to be 22.7% as calculator is limited on digits)

912 mg $\times$ 1.227 = 1119.024 mg

Round to 1120 mg

20 28.909 g

Total mass needed to be made is 29 g (28 + 1 supps of 1 g each)

Total mass of morphine sulfate needed = 29 $\times$ 5 mg = 145 mg

Displacement by morphine = 145 mg $\div$ 1.6 = 90.625 mg

Therefore, mass of base (Witepsol) = 29,000 mg − 90.625 mg = 28,909.375 mg = 28.909 g

21 1615 mL

In the recommendations section of the guideline, for routine maintenance, the initial prescription of fluids should be 25–30 mL/kg/day. Therefore, the minimum volume is 25 mL/kg/day

Calculate for this patient: 25 mL/kg/day $\times$ 64.6 kg = 1615 mL/day

22 940 mL

Protein requirements = 1.5 g/kg/day $\times$ 52.8 kg = 79.2 g/day

Each 100 mL of product contains 8.4 g of protein = 0.084 g/mL
Therefore, 79.2 g/day ÷ 0.084 g/mL = 942.8571 mL/day

23   16.4 mL/hr
295 mL ÷ 18 hours = 16.3889 mL/hour
Round to 16.4 mL/hour

24   274 mg
This patient is overweight, so the ideal body weight needs to be calculated
IBW = 45.5 + (2.3 × 4) = 54.7 kg
Then calculate the loading dose = 5 mg/kg × 54.7 kg = 273.5 mg
Round to nearest whole number which is 274 mg

25   Answer = 29.5 mL/hr
Section 4.2 of the SPC gives information on the dosing regimen to be used. As described in the question, the patient has had a loading dose so only the maintenance dose needs to be calculated
First, calculate the dose to be given per hour
1.2 mg/kg/hr × 24.6 kg = 29.52 mg/hr
Second, calculate concentration of the infusion
SPC states the vial is 10 mL so contains 250 mg aminophylline
The question states this will be diluted *to* 250 mL in sodium chloride
Therefore, 250 mg in 250 mL = 1 mg/mL (as per BNFC recommendations)
Finally, find the rate
29.52 mg/hr ÷ 1 mg/mL = 29.52 mL/hr

26   38 kg/m^2
Candidates should know the units for BMI, but this will also be provided in the answer box. From this, candidates should be able to derive the equation of BMI = weight(kg) ÷ height(m)^2
First, convert height and weight into the metric units using the BNF tables. Take care with units!
Height in m = 5′ 1″ = (5 × 304.8 mm) + 25.4 mm = 1549.4 mm = 1.5494 m
Weight in kg = 14 st 3 lb = 88.9 kg + 1.36 kg = 90.26 kg
Then calculate BMI
BMI = 90.26 ÷ 1.5494^2

If you can't find the square/power function on your calculator: BMI = 90.26 ÷ (1.5494 × 1.5494)
BMI = 37.5983 kg/m^2

27 3

Using section 4.2 of the SPC, the following formula is given when the serum digoxin level is known:
Number of vials = (serum digoxin concentration [ng/mL] × weight [kg]) ÷ 100
Rounded up to nearest vial
First ensure units for digoxin are the same
4.6 mcg/L = 0.0046 mcg/mL = 4.6 ng/mL
Therefore, vials = (4.6 × 62.8) ÷ 100 = 2.8888 = 3

28 8.8 mL/hr

3 mcg/kg/min × 78.3 kg = 234.9 mcg/min
234.9 mcg/min × 60 = 14094 mcg/hr
Infusion bags contain 160 mg in 100 mL = 1.6 mg/mL = 1600 mcg/mL
Therefore, 14094 mcg/hr ÷ 1600 mcg/mL = 8.8088 mL/hr

29 10 mg/mL

Final solution is 0.05% w/v = 0.05 g in 100 mL = 50 mg in 100 mL
The 50 mg came from 5 mL of the original solution
Therefore, 50 mg ÷ 5 mL = 10 mg/mL

30 3.158 g

Alligation can be used here
Firstly, work out how many parts each component contributes to the final product:

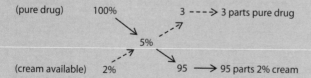

Secondly, as you know what mass of 2% cream you have, you can use this to work out the mass per part of the final product:
100 g of 2% cream ÷ 95 parts = 1.0526 g/part

Finally, use this mass per part value to work out how much salicylic acid powder is needed: 3 parts x 1.0526 g/part = 3.1578 g
Rounded to 3 decimal places = 3.158 g
Can check answer:
([mass drug in product + mass drug added] ÷ [mass of product + mass of drug added]) × 100
([2 g + 3.158 g] ÷ [100 g + 3.158 g]) × 100 = 5.0000%

31 29.2 mL
Alligation can be used here
Firstly, work out how many parts each component contributes to the final product:

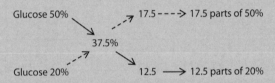

Secondly, as you know the final volume of the product (50 mL) you can use this with the total number of parts (17.5 + 12.5 parts) to work out the volume per part (mL/part)
50 mL of the final 37.5% solution ÷ 30 parts = 1.6667 mL/part
Finally, use this volume per part value to work out how much of the 50% solution is needed:
17.5 parts × 1.6667 mL/part = 29.1673 mL
Rounded to 1 decimal place = 29.2 mL
Can check answer:
50% = 50 g/100 mL = 0.5 g/mL, so in 29.2 mL there is 14.6 g glucose
20% = 0.2/mL, which makes up 20.8 mL (50 − 29.2), providing 4.16 g glucose
14.6 + 4.16 g in 50 mL = 0.3752 g/mL = 37.52 mg/100 mL = 37.52%

32 250 mcg
See section 5.2 of the SPC for the required equations
Firstly, convert serum creatinine from mcmol/L to mg/100 mL:
SeCr (mg/100 mL) = (SeCr [mcmol/L] × 113.12) ÷ 10,000 = (153 × 113.12) ÷ 10,000 = 1.7307
Secondly, work out creatinine clearance:
Ccr = (140 − age) ÷ SeCr (mg/100 mL) = (140 − 74) ÷ 1.7307 = 38.1349

Thirdly, work out the % daily loss:
% daily loss = 14 + (Ccr ÷ 5) = 14 + (38.1349 ÷ 5) = 21.627%
Then work out the maintenance dose:
Dose = peak body stores (loading dose) × (% daily loss ÷ 100) = 750 × (21.627 ÷ 100) = 162.2025 mcg
Finally, the SPC states tablets are only 66% bioavailable so this needs to be accounted for:
Tablet strength = (162.2025 ÷ 66) × 100 = 245.7614 mcg
Round to one 250 mcg tablet
The SPC indicates which strengths are available if candidates forget

33 61%
Assume 2.10 L/s is essentially 100%. Therefore, need to work out what % the 1.29 L/s is
% predicted FEV1 = (1.29 ÷ 2.10) × 100 = 61.4286%

34 340 ampoules
Section 6.6 of the SPC covers the reconstitution of this product
Each piperacillin-tazobactam 4.5 g vial requires 20 mL of sodium chloride 0.9%
Each dose also calls for two 10 mL sodium chloride amps to be used as line flushes
Thus, need four 10 mL sodium chloride ampoules per dose
Therefore, quantity to supply:
4 amps per dose × 3 doses per day × 28 days = 336 ampoules
Round to 340 ampoules
These amps come in strips of 5, question says round up

35 1329 mg
Section 4.2 of the SPC gives the following formula to use:
Iron dose (mg) = BW [kg] × (target Hb − actual Hb [g/dL]) × 2.4 + storage iron (mg)
Where the target Hb is 15 g/dL, and the storage iron is 500 mg
Remember BODMAS
Therefore, dose = 54 × (15 − 8.6) × 2.4 + 500 = 1329.44 mg

36 20.2 mmol
Section 4.4 of the SPC states that each 600 mg of product contains 1.68 mmol sodium

Therefore, each 1.2 g dose contains 3.36 mmol sodium (2 × 1.68)
Patient will receive 6 doses per day (24 hrs ÷ 4 hourly dosing)
Thus, patient will receive 6 × 3.36 mmol = 20.16 mmol sodium

37 56 tablets
Need 2 tablets per dose (2 × 480 = 960), which is equivalent to 2 tablets per dosing day
Thus, need to supply 2 × (7 × 4) = 56 tablets for the period

38 2 packs
He will take 2 tablets on five days of the week
He will take 1 tablet on two days of the week
Therefore, (2 × 5) + (1 × 2) = 12 tablets per week
Thus, 12 × 4 = 48 tablets in total
48 ÷ 28 = 1.7143 packs
So need to round up to 2 packs to ensure enough is supplied

39 10.4 mL
Need 9.5 mmol calcium (Ca^{2+}), therefore need 9.5 mmol of the calcium chloride dihydrate ($CaCl_2 \cdot 2H_2O$)
Convert the molecular mass off this directly from g/mol to mg/mmol, thus 147.01 mg/mmol
Utilise and rearrange molar equation: moles = mass ÷ molar mass → mass = moles × molar mass
Therefore, mass of $CaCl_2 \cdot 2H_2O$ needed is 9.5 mmol × 147.01 mg/mmol = 1396.595 mg
13.4% = 13.4 g in 100 mL, therefore 134 mg/mL
Thus, 1396.595 mg ÷ 134 mg/mL = 10.4224 mL

40 28.97 mg
Firstly, allocate the values for the equation
f = 0.577 (remove the minus to convert from freezing point to freezing point depression)
b = 0.576 (sodium chloride is the adjusting compound)
a requires a few steps to calculate:
5 mg in 3 mL = 1.6667 mg/mL = 166.6667 mg/100 mL = 0.1667%
Then adjust the freezing point depression value for a 0.1667% solution using the 1% value
Therefore, a = 0.1242 × 0.1667 = 0.0207

Use the numbers above in the formula given
W = (f − a) ÷ b = (0.577 − 0.0207) ÷ 0.576 = 0.9658 = 0.9658%
w/v sodium chloride
0.9658% w/v = 0.9658 g in 100 mL = 0.009658 g/mL = 9.658 mg/mL
Therefore, need 28.974 mg sodium chloride per 3 mL syringe

41 51 tablets
Miss Z needs chemoprophylaxis throughout her time in Niger
Malarone® should be started 1–2 days before entering endemic area
so 2 days will give maximum protection
Miss Z is travelling for 6 weeks and *Malarone*® should be taken
daily and continued for a week after leaving
Therefore, number of tablets needed = 2 + (6 × 7) + 7 = 51 tablets

42 275 mg
BNF monograph for paracetamol gives IV dosing in weight brackets
Dosing for 10–50 kg weight is 15 mg/kg every 4–6 hours
Therefore, dose = 15 mg/kg × 18.4 kg = 276 mg
Round to 275 mg (nearest 5 mg)

43 10 mL
BNFC monograph for paracetamol, under Pain; Pyrexia with discomfort recommends a dose of 240 mg every 4–6 hours for children
aged 4–5 years
Therefore, if there is 120 mg in 5 mL, there will be 240 mg in 10 mL

44 168 capsules
1 capsule, four times a day, for 6 weeks
Number to supply = 1 × 4 × (6 × 7) = 168

45 Answer = 112 tablets
2 tablets per dose, two doses per day, for 8 days
Tablets to supply = 2 × 2 × 28 = 112

46 Answer = 34 vials
The table in section 4.2 of the SPC states a dose of 12 mg/kg should
be used for infective endocarditis. Further down, the impaired renal
function section states the dose does not need to be adjusted until
the fourth day of treatment. Patient's with CrCl less than 30 mL/min
should receive one third of the dose daily.

3 loading doses 12 hours apart (days 1 + 2) at 12 mg/kg
Vials = 12 mg/kg × 100 kg = 1200 mg per dose × 2 doses = 2400 mg ÷ 400 mg per vial = 6 vials
Full dose on day 3 at 12 mg/kg
Vials = 12 mg/kg × 100 kg = 1200 mg ÷ 400 mg per vial = 3 vials
From day 4 onwards give one third of the full dose (note: 25 days treatment remain)
Vials = (12 mg/kg × 100 kg) ÷ 3 = 400 mg per day = 1 vial per day × 25 days = 25 vials
Therefore, total vials = 6 + 3 + 25 = 34

47 117
   ARC = 23 ÷ 350 = 0.0657
   ART = 20 ÷ 350 = 0.0571
   ARR = ARC − ART = 0.0657 − 0.0571 = 0.0086
   NNT = 1 ÷ ARR = 1 ÷ 0.0086 = 116.279
   Round up to a whole person for NNT

48 31.3%
   ARC = 27.6%
   ART = 58.9%
   ARR = ARC − ART = 27.6 − 58.9 = − 31.3%
   A risk reduction shouldn't be a negative number as this is a double negative. Therefore, the answer is 31.3% as the treatment reduces the risk of flare/disease progression

49 23.9%
   ARC = 70755 ÷ 408339 = 0.1733
   ART = 26929 ÷ 204170 = 0.1319
   RRR = (ARC − ART) ÷ ARC = (0.1733 − 0.1319) ÷ 0.1733 = 0.2389 = 23.89%
   The reference source gives a note about converting a number to a percentage should candidates forget this

50 3 vials
   Loading dose = 30 mg/kg = 30 × 13.4 = 402 mg
   Then 8 mg/kg/hr for a *further* 24 hours = 8 × 13.4 × 24 = 2572.8 mg
   Therefore 402 + 2572.8 mg total = 2974.8 mg
   Available in 1 g (1000 mg) vials so 3 vials will need to be supplied

51 4.15 mL/min
In the table, the volume (therefore dose) of the acetylcysteine to be used is banded by weight
Under the table for the first infusion, it says the dose is approximately 150 mg/kg, so you can use this to calculate the patient's weight
Weight = 9690 mg ÷ 150 mg/kg = 64.6 kg
Therefore, should use 49 mL of the concentrate of acetylcysteine
Another way of working out this volume/dose is:
The header of the table states the concentrate is 200 mg/mL
Volume to use = 9690 mg ÷ 200 mg/mL = 48.45 mL. Use the table to round up to 49 mL
Then, following the information under the table, it states that this volume of concentrate should be added to 200 mL of 5% glucose and infused over on hour
Thus, final volume = 200 mL + 49 mL = 249 mL
Therefore, rate = 249 mL ÷ 60 minutes = 4.15 mL/min

52 56 drops per minute
First, work out how many mL/minute the infusion should run at
Rate (mL/min) = 1000 mL ÷ (6 × 60) minutes = 2.778 mL/min
Candidates should know there are 20 drops per millilitre = 0.05 mL/drop
Therefore, rate = 2.778 mL/min ÷ 0.05 mL/drop = 55.56 drop/minute = 56 drop/minute

53 £918.81
Patients use one 40 mg prefilled pen every 2 weeks, meaning they will use 26 pens per year. The costs given are for two 40 mg prefilled pens, therefore incur 13 charges per year
Only need to work this out per patient
Humira® cost = 704.28 × 13 = £9155.64
Amgevita® cost = 633.60 × 13 = £8236.80
Cost saving = 9155.64 − 8236.80 = £918.84

54 0.6mL
Final product is 3 mL of a 10 mg/mL solution, which is 30 mg in 3 mL
This 30 mg comes from the 50 mg/mL solution
Volume to use = 30 mg ÷ 50 mg/mL = 0.6 mL

(Without a calculator: $50\,mg/mL$ = $5\,mg$ in $0.1\,mL$ = $30\,mg$ in $0.6\,mL$)
Can also use $C_1\,V_1 = C_2\,V_2$
Rearranged to find $V_1 = (C_2\,V_2) \div C_1 = (10\,mg/mL \times 3\,mL) \div 50\,mg/mL = 0.6\,mL$

55 83.3 mg/L
Section 5.2 of the SPC states the volume of distribution (V_d) of ceftriaxone is generally 7–12 L. Therefore, the minimum peak concentration will be achieved if the volume of distribution is greater i.e. 12 L
Estimated serum concentration = dose $\div$ V_d = 1000 mg $\div$ 12 L = 83.3333 mg/L

56 13.4 mg/L
Section 5.2 of the SPC, under Elimination, states that the elimination half-life of ceftriaxone in adults is about 8 hours. There will be approximately three half-lives to account for (24 $\div$ 8 = 3).
Therefore, need to half the serum concentration three times:
$106.8 \rightarrow 53.4 \rightarrow 26.7 \rightarrow 13.35\,mg/L$

57 105 kg
Pages 13–15 of the linked document give information on how to dose immunoglobulins by weight. The boxes on pages 14 and 15 are particularly useful here.
The first step is to calculate Mr J's ideal body weight (IBW)
IBW males = 50 + (2.3 × [height in inch – 60]) = 50 + (2.3 × [6 × 12 + 1 – 60]) = 79.9 kg
Secondly, check whether he is obese or not i.e. if actual weight is 20% greater than idea
79.9 kg × 1.2 = 95.88 kg (he is obese as he weighs 143.6 kg)
Therefore, need to use dose determining weight
DDW = IBW + 0.4 (actual body weight – IBW) = 79.9 + 0.4 (143.6 – 79.9) = 105.38 kg

58 2 g
There is a dosing table from page 18 onwards of the resource
Haemolytic disease of the newborn can be found on page 20
Dose = 0.5 g/kg = 0.5 g/kg × 4.2 kg = 2.1 g
Round to nearest gram = 2 g

59 £498,233

First calculate how many packs of medicine per year: 365 days ÷ 28 days/pack = 13.0357 packs

Round up to 14 packs (0.0357 packs is 0.9996 doses, so nearly 1 day's treatment)

Cost of omeprazole per person per year = £13.92 × 14 packs = £194.88

Cost of lansoprazole per person per year = £2.99 × 14 packs = £41.86

Cost difference for one person per year = £194.88 − £41.86 = £153.02

Therefore, cost difference for population (3256 people) = £153.02 × 3256 = £498,233.12

60 £351,104

Each patient will get 6 packs in each 6-month period (check: 365 ÷ 2 ÷ 30 = 6.0833)

Cost per person for *Truvada*® over 6 months = £355.73 × 6 = £2134.38

Cost per person for generic over 6 months = £106.72 × 6 = £640.32

Cost difference per person = £2134.38 − £640.32 = £1494.06

Cost difference for population = £1494.06 × 235 = £351,104.1

61 3 vials

First, work out the dose that needs to be prescribed. The SPC states this is 4 mg/kg every other day for 3 doses. The SPC states that once reconstituted the vials must be used within 24 hours. Therefore, need to work out number of vials per dose, then multiple by 3:

Daily dose = 49.5 kg × 4 mg/kg = 198 mg

Thus, one 300 mg vial per day (vial strength given in SPC)

Therefore, 3 vials need to be supplied

Note: if don't round up per day/dose you will get the wrong answer i.e. 4 mg/kg × 49.5 kg × 3 doses = 594 mg = two 300 mg vials

62 47.7 mL

Firstly, calculate the dose: 100 mg/kg × 18.7 kg = 1870 mg = 1.87 g

So only one vial needs to be considered here

Section 6.6 of the SPC gives more information on handling and reconstitution. This states 2 g of fosfomycin displaces 1 mL of solution.

ANSWERS

Thus, the final concentration is 2000 mg in 51 mL = 39.2157 mg/mL
So, the volume to use per dose = 1870mg ÷ 39.2157 mg/mL = 47.685 mL
Alternative method: The SPC makes a comment about a 2% volume increase if not using the whole vial, so this can be used for a slightly quicker calculation
Concentration ignoring the displacement is 40 mg/mL (2000 mg/50 mL – given in SPC)
Therefore, volume for dose = 1870 mg ÷ 40 mg/mL = 46.75 mL
2% increase for displacement = 46.75 mL × 1.02 = 47.685 mL

63 315 tablets
The dose for treating this infection is 120 mg/kg per day. The question states this is in three divided doses (TDS). Therefore, dose is approximately 40 mg/kg (120 ÷ 3 = 40)
Each dose = 40 mg/kg × 57.6 kg = 2304 mg
(Note: if 120 mg/kg/day then 120 × 57.6 = 6912 mg in 3 doses = 2304 mg per dose)
Then need to work out how many tablets per dose:
Tablets per dose = 2304 mg/dose ÷ 480 mg/tablet = 4.8 tablets
Therefore, need to assume 5 tablet per dose, which is 15 tablets per day
Finally, total tablets to supply = 15 tablets/day × 21 days = 315 tablets
There are two chances of error due to rounding at the wrong place:

- If rounding per day, not per dose:
  120 mg/kg/day × 57.6 kg = 6912 mg/day ÷ 480 mg/tablet = 14.4 = 14 tablets per day
- If rounding at the very end:
  120 mg/kg/day × 57.6 kg × 21 days = 145,152 mg ÷ 480 mg/tablet = 302.4 = 302 tablets

64 2 bottles
The BNF does not recommend a dose conversion, so the dose will still be 20 mg TDS (two 10 mg tablets TDS). The oral suspension is available as 112 mL of a 10 mg/mL concentration
Volume per dose = 2 mL (20 mg ÷ 10 mg/mL)
Volume per day = 2 mL × 3 = 6 mL
Volume over 28 days = 6 × 28 = 168 mL
Each bottle contains 112 mL, so 2 bottles will be needed

65 11.8 mL/hour
Dose 0.5 ng/kg/min × 78.6 kg = 39.3 ng/min
Concentration of infusion = 10 mcg ÷ 50 mL = 0.2 mcg/mL = 200 ng/mL
Volume per min = 39.3 ng/min ÷ 200 ng/mL = 0.1965 mL/min
Therefore, mL/hour = 0.1965 mL/min × 60 = 11.79 mL/hour

66 9 tablets
The patient is on day 3 of the regimen and is going home in the afternoon. As you are supplying the remainder of the course, you don't need to supply days 1 or 2, or the morning dose of day 3. Therefore, number of tablets needed is 9:

Day 3	Day 4	Day 5	Day 6
-	1 tablet	1 tablet	
1 tablet	1 tablet		
2 tablets	1 tablet	1 tablet	1 tablet

67 400 g
From a density of 1.25 g/mL you can determine that 1 mL of glycerol = 1.25 g
Therefore, mass of 320 mL = 1.25 g/mL × 320 mL = 400 g

68 2934.4 g
10 L = 10000 mL
Arachis oil makes up 32% of this volume = (10000 ÷ 100) × 32 = 3200 mL
From the density you can derive that 1 mL of arachis oil weighs 0.917 g
Therefore, mass needed = 0.917 g/mL × 3200 mL = 2934.4 g

69 15 mL
Candidates should know, or be able to derive from the periodic table, that the molecular formula for potassium chloride is KCl (hence the name of the product, Kay-Cee-L).
From the periodic table, the molar mass of KCl = 39.098 (K) + 35.45 (Cl) = 74.548 g/mol
This can be directly converted into millimoles: 74.548 mg/mmol

Can use these numbers to work out how many mmol/mL

Candidates should remember the following from prior study: Moles = mass ÷ molar mass

Therefore, molar concentration = 75 mg/mL ÷ 74.548 mg/mmol = 1.0061 mmol/mL

Patient needs 15 mmol per dose (30 mmol per day in 2 divided doses)

Thus, volume = 15 mmol ÷ 1.0061 mmol/mL = 14.9091 mL

70 1 bottle

Need to ensure enough for the maximum dose of 3 drops TDS, which is 9 drops per day, which is 63 drops for the treatment course (9 drops/day × 7 days)

Assume there are 20 drops in 1 mL, therefore 0.05 mL/drop (1 mL ÷ 20 drops)

Therefore, volume of drops used in the week = 0.05 mL/drop × 63 drops = 3.15 mL

Thus, only need 1 bottle for the course

71 20 g

The bag contains glucose 4% = 4 g in 100 mL fluid = 20 g in 500 mL

72 4 mL

50% = 50 g in 100 mL = 1 g in 2 mL = 2 g in 4 mL

73 62 mL

This is not as simple as working out that it is 38.75 mL (80 mg/5 mL = 16 mg/mL = 620 mg/38.75 mL)

The BNF states that doses are given as chloroquine base, and that the 80 mg/5 mL syrup is the phosphate salt, so actually contains 50 mg/5 mL of chloroquine base

Therefore, 50 mg/5 mL = 10 mg/mL = 620 mg in 62 mL

74 4 litres

1 in 10000 solution = 1 g in 10000 g of water = 1 g in 10000 mL = 1 g in 10 L

Each tablet contains 400 mg of potassium permanganate
Therefore, 1 g in 10 L = 0.1 g in 1 L = 100 mg in 1 L = 400 mg in 4 L

75   37.5 days
Two doses needed to make 100 mcg dose; this is into both nostrils; twice daily
Therefore, patient will use 2 × 2 × 2 = 8 doses per day
150 doses ÷ 8 doses/day = 18.75 days × 2 devices = 37.5 days

76   1 nanogram/mL
When you dilute 1 in 10 you make the original concentration ten times more dilute. For example, you would take 1 mL of the amphotericin suspension and dilute it to 10 mL. Serial dilutions mean you repeat this process, getting ten times more dilute each time.
Therefore, in this question you make eight serial 1 in 10 dilutions. The dilution factor = 10^8
Final concentration = 100 mg/mL ÷ 10^8 = 0.000001 mg/mL = 0.001 mcg/mL = 1 ng/mL
(Long method: 100 mg/mL ÷ 10 ÷ 10 ÷ 10 ÷ 10 ÷ 10 ÷ 10 ÷ 10 ÷ 10 = 0.000001 mg/mL)

77   Answer = 42 tablets
If the patient takes 25 mcg on one day, then 50 mcg the next day onwards on alternate days you can assume they take one 25 mcg tablet for half the days and two 25 mcg tablets for the half of the days in the 28-day period
Tablets to supply = (1 × 14) + (2 × 14) = 42 tablets

78   96 tablets
20 mg per dose with 2.5 mg tablets = 20 ÷ 2.5 = 8 tablets per dose (per week)
Number to supply = 8 tablets per week × 12 weeks = 96 tablets

79   7 prefilled pens
200 mg on day 0 = 2 pens
100 mg in 2 weeks = 1 pen
Then 100 mg every 4 weeks (week 6, 10, 14, and 18) = 4 pens
7 pens in total

ANSWERS

80 29.5 mL/min
Cockcroft and Gault formula from the BNF:

$$CrCl = \frac{(140 - age) \times weight \times constant}{SeCr}$$

Constant for men in 1.23, for women is 1.04

Therefore, $CrCl = \dfrac{(140 - 83) \times 57.6 \times 1.23}{137} = 29.4769\,mL/min$

81 140 mL
The SSP states that for every 10 mg capsule, the patient should take 2.5 mL of the oral solution. Therefore, the patient will need to take 5 mL per day (20 mg ÷ 4 mg/mL = 5 mL)
Volume to supply = 5 mL × 28 days = 140 mL
Note: the SSP talks about special container rules for this product, which mean the pharmacist can round to the nearest OP. Fluoxetine oral solution comes in 70 mL bottles, therefore the pharmacist could supply two for this patient – hence the wording of the question "require" vs "supply"

82 86.3 mL/min/1.73m^2
The Cockcroft and Gault formula should not be used here; the SPC stipulates and provides the Schwartz formula for paediatric patients. Remember to convert height from metres to centimetres
eGFR = height (cm) × 36.2 ÷ SeCr (μmol/L) = 112 × 36.2 ÷ 47 = 86.2638

83 87 capsules
125 mg = 1 capsule
Start: 1 cap × 4 doses per day × 10 days = 40 caps
Then: 1 cap × 3 doses per day × 7 days = 21 caps
Then: 1 cap × 2 doses per day × 7 days = 14 caps
Then: 1 cap × 1 dose per day × 7 days = 7 caps
Then: 1 cap × 3 doses = 3 caps
Then: 1 cap × 2 doses = 2 caps
Total = 40 + 21 + 14 + 7 + 3 + 2 = 87 capsules

84 65 mg

Section 4.2 of the SPC states that children should be dosed on body surface area. Section 6.6 gives the Mosteller formula for calculating body surface area:

$$BSA = \sqrt{\frac{Height\,(cm) \times Weight\,(kg)}{3600}} = \sqrt{\frac{126.9 \times 24.1}{3600}} = \sqrt{0.8495}$$
$$= 0.9217\,m^2$$

Loading dose = 70 mg/m^2 × 0.9217 m^2 = 64.519 mg
Round to 65 mg

85 Answer = 200 mcg

Pharmacists should know what each part of the equations mean and how to rearrange the equations. Revision on pharmacokinetics can be found in the PJ article Back to basics: pharmacokinetics: http://bit.ly/PJbasicPK

C_{pss} = Plasma concentration at steady state (i.e. target of 2.0 mcg/L)
F = Bioavailability
D = Dose
DigCl = Digoxin clearance
t = Time interval between doses
IBW = Ideal body weight

Candidates can save time if they realise that 50.1 kg is not overweight, so don't need to calculate IBW. IBW in this case is the same as her weight: 45.5 + (2 × 2.3) = 50.1 kg

Non-heart failure DigCl (L/hr) = (0.06 × creatinine clearance [mL/min]) + (0.05 × IBW [kg])
Non-heart failure DigCl = (0.06 × 27.6) + (0.05 × 50.1) = 4.161 L/hr

Need to rearrange C_{pss} equation to find D. Also, F becomes 1 (due to 100% bioavailable IV)
Thus, $D = (C_{pss} \times [DigCl \times t]) \div F = (2.0 \times [4.161 \times 24]) \div 1 = 199.728$ mcg

86 7 minutes

Under status epilepticus, the BNF recommends a maximum rate of 100 mg/minute
Therefore, rate = 680 mg ÷ 100 mg/minute = 6.8 minutes

ANSWERS

87   62 mg
     The BNF states that those who are 75 years of age or older and not
     undergoing PCI should be given a dose of 750 mcg/kg BD
     Therefore, dose = 750 mcg/kg × 82.6 kg = 61950 mcg = 61.95 mg
     Round to 62 mg

88   3 tablets
     35 mg elemental iron per tablet × 2 tabs per dose × 3 times daily
     dosing = 210 mg iron per day
     Ferrous fumarate 200 mg tablets contain 65 mg elemental iron
     Therefore, 210 mg per day ÷ 65 mg per tablet = 3.2308 tablets per
     day
     Round to 3 whole tablets
     (Question doesn't state decimal places, so give a whole number, and
     iron tablets are very difficult to split)

89   187.5 mL
     8 in 10 = 80% (8 g in 10 mL = 80 g in 100 mL)
     Therefore, can use $C_1 V_1 = C_2 V_2$
     Rearranged to find $V_1 = (C_2 V_2) \div C_1 = (3\% \times 5000 \text{ mL}) \div 80\% =$
     187.5 mL
     If not comfortable with $C_1 V_1 = C_2 V_2$ there is a long-hand method:
     Final product = 3% w/v = 3 g in 100 mL = 15 g in 500 mL = 150 g in
     5000 mL (5L)
     This 150 g need to come from the 8 in 10 acetic acid solution
     8 in 10 = 8 g in 10 g (10 mL water/aqueous solution) = 0.8 g/mL
     Therefore, volume needed = 0.8 g/mL × 150 g = 187.5 mL

90   0.0072 ppm
     Concentration of Lead (Pb) is 7.2 nanograms per gram
     7.2 ng/g = 7.2 mcg/1000 g = 7.2 mg per 1,000,000 g = 0.0072 g per
     1,000,000 g = 0.0072 ppm

91   8.1 mg/L
     You are looking for the highest concentration at 6 hours, which
     means the least amount of amount of amikacin has been cleared at
     this time point. Using a half-life of 3 hours means it takes 3 hours
     to clear 50% of the drug, whereas using a half-life of 2 hours means
     it only takes 2 hours to clear 50% of the drug. Therefore, using a
     half-life of 3 hours will give you the lowest clearance and therefore
     the maximum levels

Number of half-lives to consider: 6 hours ÷ 3 hours per half-life = 2 half-lives
Estimated level = 32.3 mg/L ÷ 2 ÷ 2 OR 32.3 mg/L ÷ 2^2 = 8.075 mg/L

92 90 mg

Firstly, need to calculate the total daily dose of morphine this lady is receiving
Daily morphine = 2 × 60 + 2 × 30 = 180 mg per day
Using the equivalent doses of morphine sulfate and diamorphine hydrochloride given over 24 hours table in this section of the BNF, candidates should be able to determine that the total daily dose of subcutaneous morphine would be 90 mg

93 12 mL

Candidates should know that the breakthrough dose for strong opioids should be one-tenth to one-sixth of the total daily amount of the regularly dosed opioids (includes regularly dose immediate release opioids e.g. QDS oxycodone and modified-release opioids)
This information is also available in the prescribing in palliative care section at the front of the BNF
First, calculate the total daily opioid dose = 60 × 2 = 120 mg of oxycodone
You want to calculate the smallest rescue dose, one-tenth is smaller than one-sixth
Therefore, rescue dose = 120 mg ÷ 10 = 12 mg
Finally, the *OxyNorm*® is 5 mg/5 mL = 1 mg/mL, so need 12 mL to get the 12 mg dose

94 10 mg patch

Pages 12 to 14 in the linked resource are the most useful here
Firstly, use Equation 1: Levodopa Equivalent Daily Dose (LEDD) = (A + B) × 0.55
A: 50 mg four times a day = 50 × 4 = 200 mg
200 mg MR at night = 200 × 0.7 = 140 mg
A = 340 mg
B: not on these medicines
B = 0
Therefore, LEDD = (340 + 0) × 0.55 = 187 mg

Then use Equation 2: Rotigotine patch dose = LEDD ÷ 20 = 187 ÷ 20 = 9.35 mg

Prescribing information says to round to nearest 2 mg, therefore 10 mg closer than 8 mg

95 1.49 mL/hour

Convert propofol concentration: 1% = 1 g in 100 mL = 1000 mg in 100 mL = 10 mg/mL

Calculate dose needed per hour: 0.3 mg/kg/hour × 49.8 kg = 14.94 mg/hour

Then work out volume per hour: 14.94 mg/hour ÷ 10 mg/mL = 1.494 mL/hour

96 78 g

In this question you're looking to work out the *weight of the substance*, which is clove oil, so the formula should be rearranged:

Weight of substance = specific gravity × weight of equal volume of water

Specific gravity is given in the question: 1.04

The weight of equal volume of water: approximately 75 g (75 mL of water being substituted)

Therefore, weight of clove oil = 1.04 × 75 = 78 g

97 100 tablets

500 mL of a 500 mg/5 mL suspension = 50,000 mg in 500 mL

50,000 mg in total ÷ 500 mg per tablet = 100 tablets

98 2220 MBq

Time difference between 07:00 and 13:00 is 6 hours. The half-life of Tc99m is 6 hours. Thus, can assume one half-life passes in this time. Therefore, radioactivity at the start time can be assumed to be twice as much of that at the end time

Radioactivity at 07:00 = 30 mCi × 2 = 60 mCi

Convert to Bq: 1 mCi is 37 MBq, so 60 × 37 = 2220 MBq

99 200 g

The BNF information on topical steroids has a table of how much cream or ointment should be needed for specific body parts for two weeks of once daily dosing. The patient is using the ointment twice daily so the amount needed should be doubled to 200 g (100 g × 2)

This product available in 100 g packs, so can supply the exact amount

100 2060 mg
You need to make a 3% excess on 100 g, so the final mass will be 103 g
The BNF entry for this product states that salicylic acid makes up 2% of the product
Therefore, 2% of 103 g = (103 ÷ 100) × 2 = 2.06 g = 2060 mg

Index